# CONTEMPORARY KINESIOLOGY:

## An Introduction to The Study of Human Movement in Higher Education

### John M. Charles

**MP**

**Morton Publishing Company**
925 W. Kenyon Avenue, Unit 12
Englewood, Colorado  80110

*To my "universal" parents,*
*Frank Stanley and Mary Barbara Charles.*
*Just as the universal joint of a sailboard*
*always provides a sound and secure anchor for the mast,*
*even while allowing it to lean where it will*
*and fall if it must, so have they nurtured me.*
*I am very grateful.*

# TABLE OF CONTENTS

# INTRODUCTION

The topic of this book is kinesiology, the academic study of human movement. Throughout the text the term *kinesiology* refers to the contemporary study of human movement in higher education. The term *physical education* is used only when it serves the more accurate historic purpose of describing programs of study that existed before the 1989 American Academy of Physical Education resolution described in detail in Chapter 1. In accordance with that resolution, a distinction is made between the study of kinesiology at the university level and physical education as it currently exists in the school system from kindergarten through 12th grade. This book is both contemporary and futuristic in that:

1.   It is the first introductory text to implement the 1989 decision of the American Academy of Physical Education to make *kinesiology* the one nationally recognized descriptor for the academic study of human movement.

2.   It responds to recent concerns about fragmentation of the field through overspecialization, by presenting the skills and knowledges of kinesiology as a comprehensive, cross-disciplinary synthesis of academic approaches.

3.   It places the study of human movement on a historical continuum from the traditions of physical education in the past to the professional and disciplinary future of kinesiology.

The breadth and comprehensiveness of the contemporary study of human movement exposes students to the range of skills and knowledge that constitute the liberal arts and sciences. Regardless of the underlying mission of a given kinesiology department, the liberal arts paradigm within which this synthesis is presented is universally applicable. The skills and knowledge derived from this liberal arts program of study are as valuable to the student concentrating in kinesiology in a professional school or education department as one who is attending a liberal arts college.

The key concepts contained in this book are:

▶ redefinition of the field of kinesiology using the most recent and up-to-date information available.

▶ reconsideration of the human movement focus of kinesiology, expanding beyond the traditional primary emphasis on sports-related physical activity to incorporate all forms of human movement.

- reappraisal of the relationship of the physical experience and its intellectual dimensions in the context of higher education.
- reorganization of the body of knowledge to emphasize the unifying features of the cross-disciplinary study of human movement.
- relocation of this body of knowledge within a liberal arts paradigm.
- realignment of the essential skills and knowledge that should underlie the study of human movement into three premises of kinesiology.
- reexamination of the promise of kinesiology in the 21st century from the perspective of its historical context. This involves pointing out evolving disciplinary implications and expanding professional applications.

In today's marketplace this is a qualitatively different text. It keeps the big picture in mind even as students delve into more specialized subareas of knowledge. It is grounded in a program of study that traditionally was based in the concepts of physical education but that has become much broader in its cross-disciplinary scope and professional mission. The breadth of its scope is attributable in part to its expansion to all forms of human movement throughout the lifespan (see chapter 1) and also to the context of higher education and the liberal arts model that promotes balance among the humanities, social science and natural science approaches to the field (see chapter 2). Thus, Part I introduces the liberal arts *paradigm* of kinesiology as its academic structure and framework in higher education.

Part II addresses the *premises* of kinesiology, or the bases for understanding kinesiology: a philosophy of action, the science of movement, and an appreciation of humans moving. Integrated within each fundamental content area are skills that are basic to liberal learning and essential for success in tomorrow's world (see chapter 3). The analytical skills of philosophy permit kinesiology students to develop principles of action, to distinguish priorities, to reach logical conclusions, to appreciate movement aesthetically, and to understand and implement ethics (chapter 4). Too frequently, introductory texts have contributed to fragmentation of the field by presenting the social science and natural science facets as separate subareas of study. To counteract this tendency, the physical law and biological science of kinesiology are introduced from interdisciplinary perspectives (chapter 5).

In chapter 6 a tradition of artificially subdividing the study of moving and being into distinct discrete academic compartments is replaced by more inclusive emphasis upon established social science disciplines and on pertinent knowledge at their intersections. For example, social psychology, the study of personality and culture and social anthropology are discussed as integrative approaches that may help students better understand individual, group, and cross-cultural manifestations of movement. The chapter concludes by offering alternative ways for students to appreciate physical activity. This entails melding perspectives of the natural and social sciences with the understanding of the humanities. In doing so, movement is better understood as a creative process and as a performing art. Just as artificially induced boundaries segregate academic knowledge (often to the detriment of the larger venture), so the experience of physical activity frequently is severed from its intellectual dimensions. Here, in contrast, the physical experience is integrated into the study of human movement as a form of applied kinesiology.

In the final part of this book, the *promise* of kinesiology is assessed by extrapolating it from historically significant evolutionary trends. Chapter 7 focuses upon the historical ideas, trends, events, and people that have influenced the study of human movement throughout time. Chapter 8 uses trend analysis from the past to envision the kinesiology curriculum of the 21st century and to analyze the professional promise of the field for students emerging from kinesiology concentrations now and in the future.

*Contemporary Kinesiology* offers a fresh approach to the study of a rapidly changing field. In addition to the college classroom, this book is appropriate for groups such as:

➤ educators and administrators offering instruction in physical activity for people of every age, physical condition, and talent level.

Curricular relevance and centrality are perennial issues in education. In a milieu of competing demands for priority, physical activity must be seen not only as an antidote to the generally poor physical condition of American children, but also as an integral feature of the educational enterprise. The diversity of approaches outlined in this book are are flexible enough to be incorporated into programs designed for target populations other than college students. The academic core and intellectual challenge of contemporary kinesiology give credibility and a sense of worth to programs based on its tenets (which may become critical factors in decisions to implement or terminate various forms of physical activity instruction).

➤ professionals in the private sector providing health, wellness, and fitness programs for consumer clientele.

In an increasingly sophisticated marketplace, providing remedies for obesity, distress, and disease may not alone guarantee success.

*Empowerment through understanding is the key to success in the proactive health industry.* Consumers want to understand psychosomatic disorders, physiological functioning, and their short-term goals and long-term purposes. Through the information in this book, professional practitioners will gain awareness of the scope of the study of human movement and how and where this knowledge can be implemented in the career field.

> ▶ individuals who want to be better informed about their own participation in physical activity.

For those whose exposure to literature about physical activity has been limited to books presenting techniques to enhance their performance, a text that informs them of the cutting edge of kinesiology may come as a welcome surprise. Individuals seeking not only to engage in, but also to *understand*, physical activities will find this book to be a valuable starting point for evaluating and enhancing their personal performance. *Contemporary Kinesiology* presents an overview of ways in which human performance may be studied, and it guides the reader toward more specialized sources in each subject area within this emerging field, through Suggestions for Further Reading at the end of each chapter.

> ▶ human movement professionals seeking to improve the quality of their service.

*Contemporary Kinesiology* seeks to redress the current imbalance between technical and critical/reflective competencies in the human movement professions. After an exhaustive analysis of practices in the biophysical, behavioral/sociocultural, and pedagogical domains of the field, Janet Harris (1993) concluded, "We must encourage greater emphasis on critical/reflective professional competencies while at the same time not losing sight of technical ones. Blending both is assumed to lead to maximal professional excellence" (p. 406). During her invited address at the prestigious 1992 Amy Morris Homans Lecture to the National Association for Physical Education in Higher Education, Harris echoed the basic premise of this book. *Contemporary Kinesiology* seeks to identify critical/reflective (and technical) competencies, to develop "more humane, creative and conscious practitioners" (p. 406).

# REFERENCE

Harris, J. C. (1993). Using kinesiology: A comparison of applied veins in the subdisciplines. *Quest, 45*(3),389–412.

# The
# Contemporary
# Kinesiology
# Paradigm

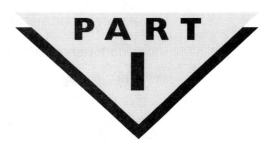

The first part of *Contemporary Kinesiology* is designed to dispel the perplexity of the academic community by thoroughly examining the meaning, focus, and structure of the study of human movement. In the first chapter, changes that have taken place in the field during the last 30 years are linked to the search for the designation of a suitable title. This is followed by examining the scope of the central focus of the field: human movement. The second chapter presents a critical analysis of the changing nature of higher education and the ways in which the field of kinesiology is responding to this evolution by gravitating toward a liberal arts format.

*University departments involved in the scholarly study of
human movement are crossing the bridge from traditional
physical education to contemporary kinesiology.*

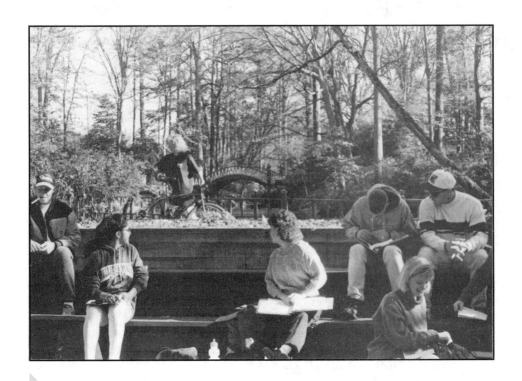

*"Therefore, be it resolved that the American Academy of Kinesiology
and Physical Education recommends that the subject matter core content
for undergraduate baccalaureate degrees related to the study
of movement be called Kinesiology, and that baccalaureate degrees
in the academic discipline be titled Kinesiology." (1989)*

# The Definition of Kinesiology

Kinesiology is more than a new name for an old field. It is the preferred designation for the scholarly study of human movement in higher education. The American Academy of Kinesiology and Physical Education (AAKPE), a distinguished group of 125 individuals selected from the profession for their outstanding contribution to the field, have chosen this title, as have the many faculty members in higher education who are replacing the departmental title of Physical Education with Kinesiology. The AAKPE resolution that put the official stamp of approval on the choice of *kinesiology* as the descriptor for the field of study was passed at the business meeting of the Academy, April 19, 1989,

*Whereas, the number and diversity of descriptors of academic programs and administrative units related to the study of human movement is now in excess of 100, and;*

*Whereas, the basic conceptual framework of this body of knowledge differs from university campus to campus, and;*

*Whereas, a multitude of degree titles, program names, and administrative rubrics has produced confusion regarding the nature of the study of movement, even among academicians who work in the field, and;*

*Whereas unanimity in description and a nationally accepted definition of the body of knowledge would provide a stronger sense of purpose, higher visibility in the academic community, and a greater understanding of the discipline by the public;*

*Therefore, be it resolved that the American Academy of Physical Education recommends that the subject matter core content for undergraduate baccalaureate degrees related to the study of movement be called Kinesiology, and that baccalaureate degrees in the academic discipline be titled Kinesiology.*

*The American Academy of Physical Education encourages administrative units, such as departments or divisions, in which the academic study of Kinesiology is predominant, to adopt the name Kinesiology. Finally, in any situation in which an administrative unit feels comfortable in describing the totality of its components by the title of the body of knowledge, the Academy recommends that this descriptor be Kinesiology. (American Academy of Kinesiology and Physical Education, 1990)*

In the footnote that accompanied this historically significant statement, the purpose of this resolution was defined as: "to give description to an academic discipline" (p. 124). By identifying a common name and focus, the Academy fulfilled its purpose, of selecting a title under which the field can unite.

This statement by the Academy brings to fruition an initiative begun a century ago by Thomas Denison Wood (1894), Director of Hygiene and Physical Training at Stanford University, and reiterated by groups of scholars in the 1950s, such as Eleanor Metheny, Camille Brown, and Rosalind Cassidy. It was continued in the 1960s by the disciplinary movement spearheaded by Franklin Henry (1964), which led to a groundswell of opinion within the field in ensuing decades, culminating in Karl Newell's (1990) proposals to change the name.

As long ago as 1893, Wood suggested, in his address to the International Congress of Education, that "the term physical education is so misleading, and even misrepresented, that we look for a name which shall represent fairly the real idea of the science" (p. 621). Recognizing that a schism was developing between disciplines purporting to study human movement, Henry (1964) stated: "There is an increasing need for the organization and study of the academic disciplines herein called physical education. As each of the traditional fields of knowledge concerning man becomes more specialized, complex, and detailed, it becomes more differentiated from physical education" (p. 32). His proposal was that physical education should reclaim the scholarly study of human movement: "If the academic discipline of physical education did not already exist, there would be a need for it to be invented" (p. 33).

Henry's proposal sparked 30 years of debate between supporters of this "disciplinarization" approach and those who preferred a traditional vocational or performance approach to physical education. During the course of this dialogue, changes in the structure and purpose of higher education concentrations pointed the way to the modern approach to kinesiology. In many instances, academic departments distanced themselves from that old ally in human performance, athletics. The Fisher Bill, passed in California in 1961, accelerated this separation by differentiating academic and nonacademic curricula in higher education. Subsequently, athletic departments hired coaches with expertise in their sports, but teacher certification could evolve only from academic departments. Consequently, physical education was redefined. Physical education departments eventually were able to change their status by showing that their programs come from the sciences, history, philosophy, psychology, and sociology.

The nature of the professional field also has become more diverse. The singular mission of teacher training, popular throughout the century, has been augmented. Preparatory programs premised upon one vocation are being replaced by those offering suitable scholarly preparation for employment in a wide range of movement professions (all careers requiring an understanding of human movement).

In this post-modern period, characterized by experimentation and questioning of time-worn principles, universities seem more willing to countenance nontraditional, cross-disciplinary programs in their curriculum. The recent appearance of programs such as American Studies, Public Policy, International Studies, and Honors and Experimental Studies on campuses across the nation set a precedent for including the scholarly study of human movement.

Recognizing these trends, the Academy (AAKPE) brought closure to the debate by selecting the name *kinesiology* to describe the study of human movement in the United States. The challenge awaiting the field of kinesiology as it enters the 21st century is to agree not only upon the name but also upon its focus and structure. Recent lively debates in *Quest*, the journal of the National Association for Physical Education in Higher Education, suggest that, although a consensus is emerging that Kinesiology is a suitable name for the broad-based study of human movement, the intellectual study of physical activity has become overspecialized and fragmented. This issue can be addressed by reformulating the study of human movement as a series of interrelated concepts integrated through a liberal arts perspective.

## FROM PHYSICAL EDUCATION TO KINESIOLOGY

Until recently, the title Physical Education had beaten back numerous challenges to its sovereignty and had survived as the preferred descriptor of the field of study. The reign of this title throughout the echelons of higher education is now at an end. If the trend documented by Brassie and Razor (1989) in *A National Survey of the Changing Structure and Names of Health, Physical Education, Recreation and Dance (HPERD) in Higher Education* continues into the 21st century, most programs of study will have adopted a title other than Physical Education by then. In the 1980s, 23% of these departments (119 of the 526 responding departments) changed names. Another 17% reported considering a change in the title of the department. Like a gathering wave, the move away from the traditional designation is gaining impetus.

## WHY NOT PHYSICAL EDUCATION?

A consensus seems to be forming in higher education that Physical Education is no longer the most appropriate descriptor, primarily because the field is undergoing a curriculum metamorphosis in the latter part of the 20th century. The title Physical Education fails to adequately describe either the focus of study or the change in approach. The field has been shifting gradually toward a more scholarly, research-oriented, disciplinary approach since Franklin Henry's initiatives. Thirty years later the reality of kinesiology is far removed from the image of physical education.

Despite the best efforts of physical educators bent on changing the image but keeping the name, the stereotypes of physical education continue to confound the academic enterprise. The obstacles in the way of salvaging the name but changing public perception of the field may be summarized as:

1. *High school hangover*. Many people think they know what physical education is because they took gym in high school. In reality, few kindergarten through 12th grade physical education programs involve more than physical activity and health. The curriculum rarely includes the intellectual domains of human movement. Consequently, the tendency in academic circles is to dismiss any program carrying the title Physical Education as being essentially practical, perhaps even recreational, and certainly peripheral to the university's intellectual mission.

2. *Jock haven*. Too often in its checkered history, physical education has been a favored concentration for college athletes. Of course, those who excel in athletic performance naturally gravitate toward the department that studies human movement. Furthermore, many student-athletes are exceptional individuals who have the renaissance quality of excelling in all spheres of learning. Unfortunately, the cynical perception of physical education too frequently is that it is a safe haven for scholarship athletes who cannot handle the rigors of simultaneously participating in sport and a challenging college major. This stereotype has been bolstered by the coincidence of teacher-coaches populating physical education departments in the past. The priority of these individuals was assumed to be coaching. They were expected to "take care" of their athletes in the classroom, giving passing grades to ensure athletic eligibility regardless of these students' academic performance. Professors today generally have undivided loyalty to their chosen field, are highly educated, hold doctoral degrees, and are as vigorous and rigorous in their research and scholarship as their colleagues in other departments across the university campus. Unfortunately, stereotypes established

over time linger despite physical education reformers' best efforts to eradicate them.

3. *Single-purpose vocational preparation.* The main purpose of physical education during the past century has been to prepare teachers for the classroom. Only recently has the focus of professional preparation broadened to encompass an array of alternative career opportunities. The one-dimensional stereotype persists to the detriment of any professional preparation programs that are attempting to broaden their focus under the auspices of physical education.

4. *Misleading descriptors.* Higher education is structured territorially. Departments focus on discrete areas of knowledge using unique methods of inquiry. The intellectual territory claimed by disciplines both defines and limits their scholarly horizons. The word "physical" stakes a claim to constraining boundaries. In a culture in which dichotomous models are popular, "physical" may be counterimposed against "intellectual" or "mental" and even "spiritual." To retain a title suggesting to many people that the study of human movement is not intellectual would be illogical and counterproductive. Department faculty would be wise to retain a title only if its symbolic advantages outweigh its negative connotations (as in the case of history, which implies a male bias but does not in fact neglect the evolution of herstory). Whereas the word "physical" is misleading and limiting, the appendage "education" is unnecessary and redundant. A student obviously goes to a university to be educated, so most disciplines forego the nicety of tacking "education" onto the end of their departmental title (e.g., Music Education). Furthermore, including "education" in the title may reinforce the archaic but popular notion of one-dimensional vocational preparation.

Physical Education is not the best title for the study of human movement. Because it is too laden with stereotypes to redeem and too entrenched in public misperception to reform, the AAKPE clearly was justified in recommending a change.

## WHY KINESIOLOGY?

Since the dawning of the realization that the title Physical Education is beyond salvaging, an array of alternative names has been considered and, in some cases, adopted. Prior to the 1989 AAKPE resolution, Kinesiology was not always the chosen name. "Exercise," "sport," "fitness," and "human movement" were popular, often legitimized with the modifier "science" or "studies" or, less frequently "arts."

The dialogue that is taking place in the United States during the latter part of this century is being mirrored worldwide. In Europe,

Physical Education generally has fallen into disfavor as the title for the field because it is "not only partially inadequate for identifying our professional endeavors within the educational system, but also completely inadequate for identifying our disciplinary activities" (Bouchard, 1974, p. 120). A range of alternatives has been tried, and in some cases found lacking. In France, exotic terms such as Anthropocinétique, Homokinetics, Anthropokineticology, and Gymnologie have been proposed along with more classic denominators such as Sport Science(s), Human Movement Science(s), Human Kinetics, Kinesiology, and Kinanthropology. In his proposal, which favored the latter term, Renson (1989) also described the ascendancy of Sportwissenschaft (Sport Science) in Germany and Human Movement in Britain and the emergence of Movement Sciences in the Netherlands.

The quandary facing faculties determined to jettison "physical education," but confronted by a plethora of alternative titles, is: What rationale should govern the choice of name? Newell, a leading advocate for the title Kinesiology, described the factors that should be taken into consideration when selecting a name. If followed closely, they would eliminate many contenders from consideration and point the way toward Kinesiology as the preferred term in the United States. He suggested (Newell, 1990) that the title should have the following qualities:

▶ *It should be representative of the field of study*. This criterion effectively eliminates titles that include facets of the focus of study, such as exercise, fitness, sport, health, leisure, recreation, and play, but do not embrace all aspects of the study of human movement. On the other hand, an umbrella term such as Kinesiology would not be appropriate for a department with a partial and exclusionary focus. Similarly, qualitative modifiers such as "arts" and "sciences" should be invoked only if they accurately circumscribe the department's focus of inquiry. "Kinesiology" is both broad and neutral, allowing its practitioners to study all aspects of human movement from the perspectives of the arts and sciences.

▶ *It should be intuitively meaningful to academia and society*. Unlike many of the improvised proposals, Kinesiology may seem valid and familiar to the college community and the general population, as it has been associated with the study of physical activity for at least a century. During that time, use of the term narrowed as kinesiology became a specialized subfield. In the 1970s, Biomechanics emerged to supersede Kinesiology as a descriptor for specific study of the mechanics of human movement. Since that time, Kinesiology has assumed a broader meaning in higher education.

- *It should have obvious academic linkage.* Whereas many of the proposed names seem to lack the form and focus of traditionally constituted departments, Kinesiology nestles snugly between social sciences such as Sociology, Psychology, and Anthropology and its closest neighbor among the life sciences, Biology.

- *It should be brief.* Patchwork titles designed to be all-inclusive, combining several areas of study into one long department name, tend to be unwieldy. Linking disparate areas of knowledge may not be feasible. Likewise, terms defining the mission of the department, such as Movement *Education*, Sports *Studies*, and Exercise *Science*, detract from titular streamlining. One word covering all the bases is preferable.

- *It should be unique.* Critical to the survival and growth of a department, particularly during a period of recessionary consolidation of programs in higher education, is that a field of study be perceived as unique and important to the university. If a title were to suggest that the study of human movement were linked, and even subordinate, to another established department, such as Kinanthropology, Sport Psychology, or Sport Sociology, it could be subsumed by that department. A unique title such as Kinesiology might allow a department to remain independent and intact.

## KINESIOLOGY: THE MOST VIABLE TITLE

The ultimate criterion in selecting the name for a university department, and for an entire field of study, is the accuracy with which the choice invokes its roots, its mission, its focus of study, and its methods of inquiry. The roots represent the history and forces that have guided the evolution of the study of human movement. The mission is the overarching purpose of the program of study. The focus of study is human movement concepts, and the methods of inquiry are the scholarly approaches selected to develop understanding of them. When measured against each of these definitional tests, Kinesiology is the most viable choice of title for the study of human movement in higher education.

## ROOTS

In their historical, anthropological, and semiological analysis of the cultural construction of kinesiology, Slowikowski and Newell (1990) traced the root word *kin* back to sixth century B. C. Greece. In the *Iliad*, Homer incorporated the three letters *k-i-n* in various verbs connoting action (e.g., walk, shake, move, budge, come, stretch, ambush). Similarly, the suffix -*logy* is a modern derivation of ancient Greek words denoting "the study and description of." The marriage of *kin* and *ology* is appropriate for a field of study that reflects the holistic traditions of Periclean Athens.

## MISSION

Slowikowski and Newell (1990) suggested that "kinesiology has been appropriated to symbolize integration and wholeness" (p. 291). Just as the term draws on ancient Greek terminology, it also invokes the cultural heritage of a period characterized by *arete* (a focus on the all-around excellence of human beings), *kalos kagathos* (twin concerns for physical beauty and moral character) and the golden mean. The well balanced, active, but reflective lifestyle espoused during that period resonates well with the integrative intent of modern-day kinesiology. Alarmed at the disintegration of the field of study caused by the insularity of specialization, a growing group of scholars suggests that the time has come for greater cooperation, collaboration, and integration as a true community of scholars. Kinesiology, with its historical ramifications of Greek holism, becomes not only the title for the department that studies human movement but also a banner signifying integrative collaboration. Slowikowski and Newell (1990) perceived the adoption of Kinesiology as a universal label for the field as symbolic of a redefined mission, new boundaries, and novel openings for interpretation (many of which are explored in this text): "The commitment by departments of kinesiology to diverse cultural, educational, scientific, and cross-disciplinary forces can be construed as a post-modern shift toward a global future for the field and for those whom we serve" (p. 289).

## FOCUS OF STUDY

The focus of study is clarified through the root meaning of kinesiology. It is the study of human movement. The umbrella term covers an array of concepts defined by the American Academy of Kinesiology and Physical Education (1990) as "(1) energy, work, and efficiency, (2) coordination, control, and skill, (3) growth, development, and form, (4) culture, values, and achievement" (p. 104). In a liberal arts context, these concepts are embedded in the humanities, social sciences, and natural sciences.

## METHODS OF INQUIRY

The methodological neutrality implicit in the label Kinesiology is what makes it particularly appropriate for the study of human movement from all disciplinary perspectives. The recent use of Kinesiology to narrowly define the mechanics of human motion triggered some transitional criticism from those who fear the encroachment of scientism. This application, however, is becoming archaic. Since the introduction of the term "biomechanics" to more accurately define the physics of human movement, the word "kinesiology" has been freed to take on a more universal meaning. In contemporary kinesiology the disciplinary approaches of science are joined by the social sciences and humanities.

Kinesiology covers the broad realm of all forms of human movement. This contrasts with physical education, which, in part because of its traditional alliance with athletics, has devoted most of its attention to athletic performance. Sport has been, and will continue to be, an important star in the constellation of kinesiology research. To limit the study of physical activity to athletic activity, however, would be to unwisely eliminate from the learning process categories of movement and segments of the population that do not involve sport. Physical activity serves many functions that kinesiologists may study in both *descriptive* and *prescriptive* ways.

The definitional double diamond depicted in Figure 1.1 differentiates the descriptive and the prescriptive modes of inquiry adopted within kinesiology. Description of the current state of affairs (*what is*) is undertaken by observing and applying of measurement techniques of the various disciplines that comprise kinesiology (for example, to

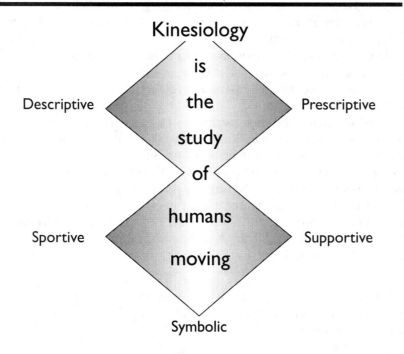

**FIGURE 1.1**
The Definitional Double Diamond of Kinesiology.

answer a question such as why and how an individual moves in a certain way). Building upon this information using empirical data and inferential logic, the kinesiologist can proceed to prescribe *what might be* (for example, how an individual could improve performance without risking injury). The modes of study in kinesiology thus, consist of analysis leading to synthesis.

In the lower diamond of Figure 1.1, distinctions are made between the types of movement that are the subject of scrutiny in kinesiology. This typology is one way of conceptualizing the multifaceted nature of the phenomenon of human movement:

1. *Sportive movement* refers to athletic activity. The primary emphasis is skill-related physical activity.

2. *Symbolic movement* is physical activity that expresses thoughts and feelings through the symbolic medium of the body. The main emphasis is physical expressivity.

3. *Supportive movement* is physical activity of a functional nature necessary to support a certain lifestyle. The major emphasis is health-related physical activity.

The separation of one subdomain of human movement from the other, for the purpose of appreciating each more fully, does not mean they are mutually exclusive. Actually, an essential feature of this paradigm of types of human movement is its integrative inclusiveness.

The diagrammatic continuum in which one line joins all three categories of movement visually reinforces the concept that sportive, supportive, and symbolic movement blend together. Conceivably, during a given activity, an individual may move from one realm to another freely and frequently. For instance, a domestic task of a supportive nature such as housecleaning, which starts as a chore, might become a form of symbolic expression, perhaps even a sportive game. Practicing an athletic skill, which is basically sportive in nature, becomes supportive when an athlete is recuperating from injury, and symbolic to the extent that players express their feelings through their actions. Dance is essentially a form of symbolism through the expressivity of the body, but for the professional dancer it is a career, with supportive ramifications and, in many competitive art forms strongly influenced by dance (such as Olympic figure skating, synchronized swimming, and rhythmic gymnastics), the main focus of movement is sportive.

## SPORTIVE MOVEMENT

Sportive movement designates athletic movements central to sport and play. These may involve varying levels of vigor and may evoke both fine and gross motor skills.

Sport is organized, competitive activity played at every level, by people of all ages with varying levels of seriousness. The competition in sport may take a variety of forms, including:

| | |
|---|---|
| 1 vs. 1: | individual sports such as tennis |
| 1 vs. many: | activities such as marathon running and triathlons |
| many vs. many: | team sports such as football and basketball |
| 1 vs. standards: | competing against a distance (jumps, throws) and time (racing events, time trials) |
| 1 vs. nature: | many outdoor activities, such as rock climbing |
| 1 vs. self: | for example, to improve performance and overcome fear |

The extent of organization may fluctuate, although as a sport becomes more developed, it tends to be accompanied by more rules and regulations. High-level athletic performance is a cultural phenomenon of great public interest. Professional sports culminating in popular events such as the Olympic Games, the Super Bowl, and World Cup soccer grip the attention of nations. Kinesiology has considerable scholarly significance in sport because of the dramatic cultural impact of organized sports. Influenced by media coverage of sport and concerns for their own health, people of all ages, of every skill level, and in the full range of physical conditions are active in sports. Consequently, sportive activity has much personal significance for many students entering the field of kinesiology.

Play spans the sportive and expressive categories of movement. One can play in sport; indeed, most games start out as play. It initially is nonserious creative activity played for its own sake. As it becomes more worklike, sport may veer from play to a more utilitarian activity undertaken for rewards extrinsic to the event. The category of sportive movement encompasses not only popular modes of competitive sport but also playlike activities associated with recreational leisure, such as camping and boating.

Although sportive physical activity has captured the most attention in kinesiology, the expressive dimensions of human movement have been gaining interest. Eleanor Metheny (1954), a pioneer in the symbolic nature of movement, stated:

## SYMBOLIC MOVEMENT

*The body is the physical manifestation of the person, his mind, his emotions, his thoughts, his feelings. . . . Through its movements he expresses and externalizes the thinking and feeling which makes him a unique person. And as he moves, the very act of movement modifies and affects his thinking and feeling and being.*

As Metheny suggested, the human body is a source of symbolism. Its movement may perform twin functions of expression. On the one hand, movement is an *introspective* form of self-exploration. It provides a venue for self-discovery. Through motor activity, people define their limitations and test those limits. Physical activity is not only a venue for increasing self-awareness but also is a dimension through which each person may express creativity. The body is the instrument through which people may compose their own works of art. The creative process may be directed into compositions requiring disciplined fine motor skills, such as those necessary for brush strokes and sculpting, or the precise movements of ballet and formal gymnastics. Alternatively, creativity may be expressed in the free-flowing form of contemporary dance, certain outdoor adventure activities, or spontaneous play.

On the other hand, movement acts as an *extrospective* form of communication (to others) of one's inner thoughts and feelings. As contrasted with self-defining forms of introspective activity, extrospective activity is externally directed. Through extrospective activity, inner feelings may be conveyed to observers. These movement messages may be purposive or coincidental. *Purposive* forms are designed with an intended impact using predefined patterns of movement, as with much modern dance. *Coincidental* physical activity is the unintended, accidental, or subliminal expression of feelings and reactions through the medium of movement. Coincidental physical expression is part of every movement moment, ranging from the gestures and signals accompanying athletic activity to the nonverbal aspects of daily communication.

Symbolic expressivity inevitably is part of physical activity. When people move, they do so in their own unique ways with purposes and meanings of their own. Whereas self-expression may be incidental to sportive activity, it is the basis of many performing art forms such as dance. It also is an inherent aspect of daily dialogue. Words are supplemented by actions, or nonverbal signals that enhance communication. When deprived of words, human beings develop a language of the body to enable communication. Body language — the expression of interpersonal meanings through physical activity — is a form of human movement that merits more attention within kinesiology because of its significance in daily interaction.

## SUPPORTIVE MOVEMENT

As Thomas (1990) suggested, traditionally "we have shown more interest in overhand striking patterns in tennis players than in carpenters, . . . mental practice in high jumpers than in metal riveters" (p. 9). Recent diversification in the field has sought to remedy this shortcoming by actively focusing on supportive movement. Healthy physical functioning has become a major concern of kinesiology. For example, wellness, the subarea of kinesiology devoted to enhancing personal well-being, centers on supportive, not sportive, activity. The emphasis is on the level and quality of health-related exercise necessary to support a certain lifestyle rather than on skill-related performance. Contemporary kinesiology transcends the traditional physical emphasis on athletic ability to a focus upon the needs, capacities, and potential of individuals throughout their day's work and play.

## SUMMARY

During the last 30 years the study of human movement has become a full-fledged field of scholarly inquiry. It continues to develop rapidly. The title Physical Education does not adequately describe, or even introduce, the modern program. Endorsed by the American Academy of Physical Education as the preferred name, Kinesiology more accurately connotes the roots, mission, methods of inquiry, and focus of study of the field. Contemporary kinesiology is concerned with all forms of human movement. The core curriculum includes sportive, symbolic, and supportive forms of human movement phenomena. University departments involved in the scholarly study of human movement are crossing the bridge from traditional physical education to contemporary kinesiology.

## REFERENCES

American Academy of Kinesiology and Physical Education. (1990). Resolution on kinesiology. In *Academy Papers* (Vol. 23, p. 104). Champaign, IL: Human Kinetics.

Bouchard, C. (1974). Les sciences de l'activité physique: Un concept fondamental dans notre organisation disciplinaire et professionelle. *Mouvement, 9*, 120.

Brassie, P. C., & Razor, J. E. (1989). *A national survey of the changing structure and names of H.P.E.R.D. in higher education*. Reston, VA: American Alliance for Health, Physical Education, Recreation and Dance.

Henry, F. M. (1964). Physical education: An academic discipline. *Journal of Health, Physical Education and Recreation, 35* (7), 32-33.

Metheny, E. (1954). The third dimension in physical education. *Journal of Health, Physical Education, and Recreation, 25*, 27-28.

Newell, K. M. (1990). Kinesiology: The label for the study of physical activity in higher education. *Quest, 42*(3), 272-273.

Renson, R. (1989). From Physical Education to Kinanthropology: A quest for academic and professional identity. *Quest, 41*, 235-256.

Slowikowski, S. S., & Newell, K. M. (1990). The philology of kinesiology. *Quest, 42*(3), 281.

Thomas, J. R. (1990). The body of knowledge: A common core. In *Academy Papers* (Vol. 23, pp. 5-13). Champaign, IL: Human Kinetics.

Wood, T. D. (1894). Some unsolved problems in physical education In *Proceedings of the International Congress of Education of the World: Columbian Exposition* (pp. 621-623). New York: National Education Association.

# SUGGESTED READING

Adams, W. C. (1991). *Foundations of Physical Education, Exercise and Sport Sciences*. Philadelphia: Lea and Febiger.

Barrow, H. M., and Brown, J. P. (1988). *Man and Movement: Principles of Physical Education*. Philadelphia: Lea and Febiger.

Blonsky, M. (Ed.). (1985). *On Signs*. Baltimore: Johns Hopkins University Press.

Bucher, C. A. (1983). *Foundations of Physical Education and Sports*. St. Louis: C. V. Mosby Co.

Cheffers, J. T., & Evaul T. (1978). *Introduction to Physical Education: Concepts of Human Movement*. Englewood Cliffs, NJ: Prentice-Hall.

Colfer, G. R., Hamilton, K. E., Magill, R. A., & Hamilton, B. J. (1986). *Contemporary Physical Education*. Dubuque, IA: Wm. C. Brown Publishers.

Drowatzky, J. N., & Armstrong, C. W. (1984). *Physical Education: Career Perspectives and Professional Foundations*. Englewood Cliffs, NJ: Prentice-Hall.

Freeman, W. H. (1992). *Physical Education and Sport in a Changing Society*. New York: Macmillan.

Kearney, R. (1989). *The Wake of Imagination: Toward a Post Modern Culture*. Minneapolis: University of Minnesota Press.

Lumpkin, A. (1986). *Physical Education: A Contemporary Introduction*. St. Louis: Times Mirror/Mosby.

Lawson, H. A. (1984). *Invitation to Physical Education*. Champaign, IL: Human Kinetics.

Siedentop, D. (1990). *Introduction to Physical Education, Fitness and Sport*. Mountain View, CA: Mayfield Publishing Co.

Zeigler, E. F. (1990). *Sport and Physical Education: Past, Present, Future*. Champaign, IL: Stipes Publishing Co.

**2**

# The Place of Kinesiology in Higher Education

F ranklin Henry (1978), clarified the key concepts of the academic curriculum in an article in *Quest*. In that paper he reexamined the ideas he originally presented in an address to the annual meeting of the National College Physical Education Association for Men in 1964. He suggested that the academic discipline should be organized horizontally (as well as vertically) on a cross-disciplinary basis to include exercise physiology, motor learning, motor development, biomechanics, and the roles of athletics, dance, and other physical activities in the culture. Based in part on his assessment of the state of the art, a dominant model of academic physical education has evolved in higher education.

For 30 years the academic discipline has been structured along the lines Henry recommended. The Big Ten directors in the mid 1960s as well as Haag (1979), Bucher (1983), and Barrow and Brown (1988) in the 1970s and 1980s have been in general accord about the subject matter suitable to include in the core academic curriculum. These are summarized as follows:

**THE TRADITIONAL PHYSICAL EDUCATION MODEL**

**Big Ten Directors (1964):**  history and philosophy, exercise physiology, biomechanics, motor learning, sport psychology, sport and culture, and administrative theory in athletics and physical education

**Haag (1979):** sport history and philosophy, anatomy and physiology, sport medicine, sport biomechanics, sport psychology, sport sociology, and sport pedagogy

**Bucher (1983):** history, anatomy and physiology, biomechanics, psychology and sociology

**Barrow and Brown (1988):** history and philosophy, anatomy and physiology, biomechanics, motor learning, psychology, anthropology, sociology, and growth and performance

The similarity of topics chosen by this generation of leaders in the field indicates a consensus on what conceptual criteria should define the undergraduate curriculum. Thomas (1990) summarized these concepts as being:

- human anatomy/function.
- physical growth and motor development.
- biomechanical aspects of movement.
- acute and chronic effects of exercise.
- behavioral and neuromuscular control of movement.
- acquisition of motor skill.
- psychological factors in movement, exercise, and sport.
- sociocultural factors in movement, exercise, and sport.
- history/philosophy of movement, exercise, and sport.

With appropriate prerequisites from the traditional disciplines in the physical, biological, and social sciences, and the humanities, the traditional core curriculum systematically presents these nine concepts as aspects of knowledge of human movement.

## THE CONTEMPORARY KINESIOLOGY MODEL

By the 1990s the focus of the study of human movement has broadened to emphasize:

- alternative professional occupational outlets.
- the intellectual meanings and ramifications of performance and physical experiences.
- conceptual rather than disciplinary approaches to curriculum construction.
- collegial cooperation *between kinesiology professors* to avoid fragmentation of the field caused by overspecialization and *within the university* to contribute in meaningful ways to the greater endeavor of higher education.

Figure 2.1 illustrates the symbiotic interrelationships of the study of movement, physical activity experience, and professional preparation.

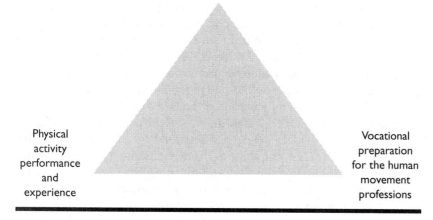

The study of human movement (sciences)
and humans moving (social sciences and humanities)

Physical
activity
performance
and
experience

Vocational
preparation
for the human
movement
professions

**FIGURE 2.1**
The Triad of Kinesiology

They are symbiotic in that, although they are separate and distinct aspects of kinesiology, they each play a vital role in defining each other.

The academic study of human movement has changed in both form and function, in part because professional opportunities are changing radically. As Krahenbuhl (1991), a university dean and contemporary higher education analyst, suggested, disciplines tend to take their shape from social evolution. As trends emerge in the culture surrounding the university, the institution typically responds:

*Late in the last century, psychology formed as a body of knowledge from various disciplines interested in the study of the mind and behavior. Early in this century, biochemistry grew out of biology and chemistry. The discipline of political science grew out of early education programs preparing high school teachers of government and academic programs in political philosophy. At the moment, cellular and molecular biology programs are being formed around the advances in biotechnology. (p. 91)*

He concluded that kinesiology is having a similar growth spurt because of the changing emphasis upon human movement in today's culture. Professional applications have curricular implications. Ellis (1990) suggested that this relationship between discipline and profession should be oriented toward refinement of the profession.

*A core curriculum should be integrated around a conceptual structure that derives its logic from the phenomena of human movement, not the cognate disciplines. It should integrate that knowledge in ways that illuminate the real problems of the professions it is designed to serve rather than reflecting the conveniences of staffing the university department with subspecialties. (p.16)*

Such a curriculum, he concluded, would encompass topics such as cell physiology/tissue system physiology, anatomy, biomechanics, neuroscience/motor control, motor learning, social psychology, anthropology of human movement, and philosophic and religious thought.

Driven by the opportunities of the marketplace and by changing perceptions of the importance of the study of supportive and symbolic movement, the core curriculum in kinesiology is changing. The reconceptualization of the field of knowledge around thematic constructs by the American Academy of Kinesiology and Physical Education in 1989 laid the groundwork for the reformulation of the core curriculum in the 1990s. Similarly, the nine concepts described by Thomas (1990) are changing subtly to an emphasis on understanding the fundamental qualities of movement rather than illuminating the parent disciplines. The contemporary kinesiology model is broadening to accept new ways of studying human movement and is prepare graduates to enter a wider array of human movement professions than was possible in the early days of exclusive emphasis upon teacher preparation. Adoption of a liberal arts approach to the study of human movement is one of the contributing factors to recent changes in the field.

The liberal arts are "liberal" in one sense in that they apply liberally to men and women of all ages and conditions. They provide universally valuable wisdom that may be generally useful in life as well as narrowly valuable in a job. A liberal education is more than a form of information gathering; it is a process of liberation from "the closing of the American mind" (as the root word "liberalis" would imply). In his review of Allan Bloom's (1987) controversial best-seller under that title, Sydney Hook (1989) listed the essential qualities of a liberal education in his proposal of what students need to know. He concluded that students should gain knowledge of:

- the body and mind.
- the world of nature.
- how society functions.
- the historical, social, and economic forces that have shaped the past and are likely to shape the future.

He also identified the skills underlying liberal education as:

- comprehension of different types and levels of discourse.
- the ability to distinguish between arbitrary and reasonable judgments of value.
- the ability to express oneself in a literate manner.
- familiarity with the scientific method.
- an understanding of evidence, relevance, and the canons of reliability and validity.

A liberal arts approach to kinesiology incorporates all of these knowledges and skills into a multifaceted focus upon the intellectual meanings of human movement and the harmonious development of mind and body.

## THE LIBERAL ARTS INSURGENCE IN PROFESSIONAL PREPARATION

The mission of any academic department depends upon the administrative unit in which it is housed. The core curriculum of each department may be expected to reflect that higher purpose. A review of *Peterson's Guide* (Von Vorys, 1990) reveals that of the 290 institutions granting graduate degrees in physical education/kinesiology, 37 (13%) are housed in liberal arts colleges, 70 (24%) in professional colleges of various names (such as Health, Physical Education and Recreation, or Allied Health), and 183 (63%) in education colleges. The wrong conclusion to draw from these demographic data is that the liberal arts approach outlined in this text is relevant only to a handful of colleges. In recent years, dramatic changes have taken place in colleges of education and professional schools. The net effect of these changes is to make a liberal arts approach to the study of human movement universally applicable at all institutions of higher learning.

Professional preparation is becoming more liberalized. Professions such as medicine, law, and business are seeking individuals with more than basic technological capability. They want to attract more comprehensively educated individuals to populate their professions. The case of the medical profession is particularly salutary for kinesiology because of the increasing intersection between the medical and movement professions. The *Journal of Medical Education* recently highlighted the shape of things to come in the 21st century. It concluded that medical undergraduate education must "encompass broad study in the humanities and in the social as well as the natural sciences" (Levy, 1988, p. 130). Within the medical field the consensus is emerging that the physician's general professional education should include a common foundation of knowledge, skills, values, and attitudes and a sound general liberal arts and science baccalaureate education. Kinesiology is an excellent undergraduate springboard to the biophysical medical and allied health professions, particularly those that concentrate on physical activity, play, and exercise as therapy.

Schools of education have undergone a similar metamorphosis in the wake of a call for reform in commission reports such as that of the Carnegie Commission 1987, the Holmes Group in 1986, and the private opinions of individual professors expressed in best-selling books such as those by Bloom (1987) and Hirsch (1987). The net effect of all of these proposals is to steer teacher preparation toward the liberal arts. According to Siedentop (1990), "Virtually every education reform document calls for more liberal arts courses for future teachers" (p. 30). The impetus begun by the Holmes Group proposal, the Carnegie Forum on Education and the Economy, and the various state department of education initiatives to improve teacher education programs will continue into the 21st century. The face of teacher education is changing dramatically, as the following Holmes Group proposals are being implemented:

▶ Teacher education programs should be more substantive and more relevant in terms of the academic subject matter to be taught.

▶ The general education preparation for teachers should be as rigorous as that required of students in the liberal arts and sciences.

▶ The subject matter background preparation for teachers should be increased in a manner consistent with the growth in knowledge in virtually all disciplines.

▶ The clinical aspects of teacher preparation programs should be more sophisticated and interspersed throughout the professional component of the program. (Smith, 1986, pp. 52–56)

In many cases, student teachers who previously would have obtained their certification to teach through a 4-year program combining academic subject matter and professional methodology courses now will complete a 4-year undergraduate degree as rigorously intellectual as any liberal arts student before proceeding to complete teacher certification requirements in a fifth year. Students wishing to teach physical education in the school system logically would be expected to declare an undergraduate concentration in kinesiology. Faculty and departments in schools of education that certify these students to teach are taking a fresh look at the subject matter constituting the study of human movement and are incorporating a liberal arts approach into their curriculum.

## THE LIBERAL ARTS INSURGENCE IN THE UNIVERSITY

To be acceptable within the university community, kinesiology must be perceived as contributing to the mission of undergraduate education in a unique and important way. Given that the liberal arts approach is becoming more universally accepted throughout higher education, the study of human movement should be consistent with liberal arts philosophy as it is interpreted and presented in the modern university. That it has remained relatively intact through the ages is a testament to the durability and resilience of the liberal arts approach to higher education. In 1852, Cardinal John Henry Newman (rector of the Catholic University of Ireland in Dublin) presented a series of discourses now compiled under the title *The Idea of a University* (1976). In the introduction to his seventh discourse, under the title, "Knowledge Viewed in Relation to Professional Skill," Newman defined liberal education and the university as follows:

*This process of training, by which the intellect, instead of being formed or sacrificed to some particular or accidental purpose, some specific trade or profession, or study of science, is disciplined for its own sake, for the perception of its own proper object, and for its own highest culture, is called Liberal Education; and though there is no one in whom it is carried as far as is conceivable, or whose intellect would be a pattern of what intellects should be made, yet there is scarcely any one but may gain an idea of what real training is, and at least look toward it, and make its true scope and result, not something else, his standard of excellence; and numbers there are who may submit themselves to it, and secure it to themselves in good measure. And to set forth the right standard, and to train according to it, and to help forward all students toward it according to their various capacities, this I conceive to be the business of a University. (p. 1)*

In 150 years, the business of the university has undergone revision, and the concept of education for its own sake has been refined, but the basic vision of Cardinal Newman still undergirds the modern liberal arts approach. The ideal of learning because knowledge is its own reward dates back through the centuries. Aristotle, who began the first book of the Metaphysics with the phrase, "All men by nature desire to know," and one of Newman's favorite sources, Cicero, who declared that "only man possesses the capacity to seek and pursue truth" are examples of this approach. Newman (1976) cited the authority of Cicero to support his own principle when he, "in enumerating the various heads of mental excellence, lays down the pursuit of Knowledge for its own sake, as the first of them."

The often cited criticism of this liberal arts approach is that it is not obviously useful in today's world. How can a graduating student emerging from a school that espouses Newman's principle — "that knowledge is not merely a means to something beyond it, or the preliminary of certain arts into which it naturally resolves, but an end sufficient to rest in and to pursue for its own sake" — expect to get a job? A liberal education is not linked directly to the job market in the narrow, vocational sense of professional competencies. This quality makes this approach to education for the real world more, not less, useful. As Pelikan (1992) suggested in *The Idea of the University: A Re-examination*, "This definition does not imply, as many of its critics and even some of its defenders have occasionally supposed, that the liberal learning which is the university's reason for being, must never produce anything useful or have any sequel or consequence; it means only that its pursuit is not to be justified principally on those grounds" (pp. 33-34).

Rather than being tied to the dictates of an ephemeral employment market or the vested interest of special interest groups (awaiting the emergence of freshly trained undergraduate students from job certification trade schools), modern universities are proudly independent. A liberal education is a liberating experience. It allows faculty and students to develop critical consciousness and cultural awareness through teaching and learning, research, and publication. Yet, liberal education is not divorced from the professions. The fundamental knowledge about human movement, considered in its broadest context, provides an invaluable foundation for professional training. In *The Choices for a University*, Levi (1969) indicted the old professional school model: "The professional school which sets its course by the current practice of the profession is, in an important sense, a failure" (p. 38). The justification for such a severe judgment is that "the professional school must be concerned in a basic way with the world of learning and the interaction between the world and the world of problems to be solved" (p. 38). His conclusion is that the evolving professional school should adopt a liberal arts approach. "Viewed in terms of its larger responsibilities, the professional school inherits and exemplifies much of the disappearing tradition of the liberal arts college. As such it represents some of the highest values in a university" (p. 39).

In summary, the liberal arts tradition based on ancient Greek and Roman precepts of learning, formulated by Newman in 1852 and reexamined by Pelikan (1992), is an enduringly valuable approach to undergraduate education. It facilitates the growth of the independent learner, one who Newman suggested, "has learned to think and to reason and to compare and to discriminate and to analyze, who has refined his taste, and formed his judgment, and sharpened his mental vision" (p. ). The liberal arts tradition is not opposed to professional training but, rather, is complementary to it, for through this approach a student may be "placed in that state of intellect in which he can take up any one of the sciences or callings I have referred to, or any other for which he has a taste or special talent, with an ease, a grace, a versatility, and a success, to which another is a stranger" (Newman, 1976, p. 6).

## THE LIBERAL ARTS INSURGENCE IN KINESIOLOGY

By its very nature, kinesiology is an ideal foundational component of the undergraduate liberal arts experience. Similarly, a kinesiology *concentration* is uniquely conducive to the implementation of a liberal arts approach for several reasons:

1. Human movement is a *universal phenomenon*. Every body moves. We all experience our bodies daily and move constantly.

Whereas the focus of some academic departments may seem removed from daily experience, human movement is central to it.

2. Physical activity is *culturally popular*. Pelikan (1992) stated, "Except perhaps for big time soccer, the university seems to have become the most nearly universal, man-made institution in the modern world" (p. 22). It is fitting that one human universal (physical activity in its broadest context, including sport) should become a major focus of the universal university.

3. Human movement is an *attractive focus*. Most students are young, energetic individuals who find the study of physical activity intrinsically rewarding. The insights they gain may be both personally and professionally satisfying.

4. The study of human movement is *the exclusive academic terrain of kinesiology*. Although other departments may focus on physical activity phenomena peripherally, only kinesiology places human movement at the center of its universe and studies it in a constellation of different ways. By integrating and magnifying discrete portions of many disciplines, the study of human movement is developed in an orderly, logical sequence. Thus, kinesiology has the advantages of:

    ▶ treating human movement phenomena as ends meriting study in their own right rather than as means to illuminating another disciplinary mode of inquiry.

    ▶ applying a holistic approach to the focus of study rather than the reductionist model often characteristic of higher education.

    ▶ allowing alternative approaches to professional preparation, leading to a multiplicity of careers.

5. Kinesiology has *multiple professional complementarity*. Multidisciplinary study of human movement produces understandings that may be parlayed into a variety of rewarding careers through further graduate study and professional preparation. As the last vestiges of narrowly focused professional preparation are eliminated from the undergraduate liberal arts major, the confining linkage of the concentration to predefined careers is expanded to lead toward a multiplicity of future vocations and avocations. The popularity of human movement phenomena, particularly sport, in society translates into a major research opportunity in higher education. The pervasiveness of participation, the plethora of information and statistics, and the cultural meanings of sport fuel a significant

research agenda. Similarly, growing cultural emphases upon symbolic and supportive movement are opening avenues of professional opportunity for kinesiology students with expertise and understanding in these areas (see chapter 8).

6. The teaching of kinesiology features *pedagogical versatility*. The horizontal (as well as vertical) structure of kinesiology allows faculty to approach human movement from diverse perspectives. (The verticality of a curriculum is determined by the narrowness of its focus and the hierarchical structure of the arrangement of knowledge.) Many disciplines are associated with one dominant method of packaging and disseminating information which may lead to a certain uniformity of teaching style. Kinesiology students, however, typically are exposed to an array of teaching styles and ways of thinking because of the range of concepts to be considered in the curriculum. Consequently, kinesiology is uniquely capable of instilling the skills of a liberal education. In each of the kinesiology classes (ranging through the humanities, social sciences, and natural sciences), students encounter differing pedagogical emphases and develop the different learning skills fundamental to liberal learning (discussed in Chapter 3).

7. The kinesiology curriculum has *conceptual universality*. Kinesiology is comparable to such new and emerging programs as American Studies and Public Policy in its conceptual bredth. Through the study of human movement, students are exposed to most of the pillars of wisdom underlying the liberal arts, found in the realms of the humanities, social sciences, and natural sciences.

8. Kinesiology has *experiential potential*. Human movement, by definition, is a dynamic phenomenon — one that can be understood through both intellectual abstraction and experience. Within the context of kinesiology, a range of experiential teaching and learning conditions can be developed. Each of these can be designed not only to educate students in the use of their bodies but also to use physical activity to illuminate the theoretical concepts that pervade the study of human movement. By stressing the symbiotic relationship of the movement experience and its study, contemporary kinesiology integrates the mind and the body in a holistic fashion, rather than separating the intellectual from the physical and relegating the latter to a lower rung on the academic ladder, which has tended to be the norm in higher education.

Kinesiology is uniquely capable of contributing to the university's function of transmitting, cultivating, and criticizing learning. The study of human movement is structured to resonate with "the common learning" of a liberal arts education. Through a comprehensive approach to the study of human movement phenomena, students absorb specialized information that will be useful in their professional futures without ever losing sight of the bigger picture. The challenge of the future for kinesiology, as a training ground for the human movement professions, can be compared to that of biology as a preparation for the medical professions. As Pelikan (1992) stated, "Human biology must be studied within the total context of biology, and those who are being prepared to apply the information and insights of human biology to the art of healing must be at home within the larger context or they will not be professionally (not to say scientifically) equal to their tasks" (p. 105).

The larger context of the liberal arts approach to kinesiology is at the heart of the mission of the modern university. It entails introducing students to certain spheres of knowledge while including a range of learning skills. Kinesiology is structured in accordance with these criteria with the aim of producing a liberally educated graduate. (In many cases, its acceptance as a credible academic unit on campus may depend upon successful implementation of this strategy.) The essential liberal arts skills and knowledges are illustrated in Figure 2.2 in the diagrammatic form of the kinesiology "umbrella."

The ribs of the umbrella represent the following liberal learning skills:

- critical thinking skills.
- scientific skills.
- quantitative skills.
- inquiry skills.
- communication skills.
- aesthetic skills.

Covering these foundations is the fabric of knowledge that covers the total undergraduate liberal arts kinesiology experiences of:

- gaining a philosophic foundation.
- acquiring scientific knowledge of human movement.
- understanding humans moving as a form of individual and socio-cultural behavior.
- appreciating humans moving as an artistic, creative, and personal experience.

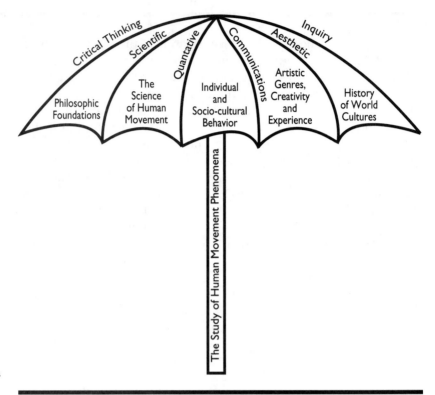

**FIGURE 2.2**
The Kinesiology Umbrella

The labels on the umbrella, from left to right:

- Critical Thinking
- Scientific
- Quantative
- Communications
- Aesthetic
- Inquiry

Canopy sections:
- Philosophic Foundations
- The Science of Human Movement
- Individual and Socio-cultural Behavior
- Artistic Genres, Creativity and Experience
- History of World Cultures

Handle: The Study of Human Movement Phenomena

inquiring into historically significant events, ideas and movements, and trends from the past that might illuminate the future.

The umbrella concept illustrates the range of skills and knowledge areas that constitute kinesiology, but it does not do justice to their interrelatedness. Each aspect of the total fabric of knowledge may combine any or all of the skills into a holistic learning experience.

## SUMMARY

Pelikan (1992) concluded that "the liberal arts provide a means for the individual to understand his or her relationship to the larger environments" (p. 105). The relevance of a liberal education in today's world is its explanatory power. Students emerge from a high-quality program having been exposed to a range of ideas and disciplinary approaches. They are equipped to think critically and to research independently. Recognizing the value of a liberal arts foundation, professional schools, including Schools of Education, increasingly are seeking individuals who have been exposed to the concepts and skills of a liberal education to populate their professions.

The evolution of the liberal arts approach to education can be traced back to Newman. More recently, Pelikan has suggested that, today, a liberal arts education has retained its initial basic features but has been modified subtly to meet the demands of the 21st century. Contemporary kinesiology has a natural affinity with the liberal arts. Human movement is a universal phenomenon with innate appeal. It is a unique focus of inquiry of considerable cultural significance. It lends itself well to the range of liberal arts concepts, values, and skills, from a multiplicity of modes of investigation. It melds the intellectual with the experiential into a holistic applied field of study. Kinesiology graduates are well prepared for the many professions that are based on human movement.

The discussion of the meanings, structure, and direction of kinesiology clearly points to the liberal arts pathway as the way to go. Factors contributing to this trend are the changing demands of the human movement professions, the new expectations of graduate schools and professional schools that offer advanced certifications, and the recent curricular evolution of undergraduate education. The human movement professions are seeking versatile individuals with a broad base of intellectual sophistication, capable of recognizing an array of options and of reacting to the challenges of the 21st century. Admission to graduate programs and advanced certification is premised upon high quality, comprehensive awareness of the multidimensional study of human movement. Undergraduate education is responding to the challenges of post-modern society by deemphasizing subject boundaries and encouraging cross-disciplinary curricular innovations. Notwithstanding their willingness to entertain initiatives such as kinesiology, the modern university is itself in a highly competitive marketplace and will insist (for reasons of self-preservation) that new programs must contribute meaningfully to the university's academic mission.

# REFERENCES

Barrow, H. M., & Brown, J. P. (1988). *Man and movement: Principles of physical education*. Philadelphia: Lea and Febiger.

Bloom, A. (1987). *The closing of the American mind*. New York: Simon and Schuster.

Bucher, C. A. (1983). *Foundations of physical education and sport*. St. Louis: C. V. Mosby Co.

Ellis, M. J. (1990). Reactions to "The Body of Knowledge: A Common Core." In *Academy Papers* (Vol. 23, pp. 13-16). Champaign, IL: Human Kinetics.

Haag, H. (1979). Development and structure of a theoretical framework for sport science. *Quest, 31*, 25-35.

Henry, F. M. (1978). The academic discipline of physical education. *Quest, 9*, 53-57.

Hirsch, E. (1987). *Cultural literacy: What every American needs to know*. Boston: Houghton-Mifflin.

Holmes Group Executive Board. (1986). *Tomorrow's teachers: A report of the Holmes Group*. East Lansing, MI: Holmes Group.

Hook, S. (1989). The closing of the American mind: An intellectual best-seller revisited. *American Scholar, 58*(1), 123-125.

Krahenbuhl, G. S. (1991). Physical education in American higher education. In *Academy Papers* (Vol. 24, pp. 89-92). Champaign, IL: Human Kinetics.

Levi, E. H. (1969). *Point of view: Talks on education*. Chicago: University of Chicago Press.

Levy, R. (1988). The impact of science on medicine. In P. T. Marsh (Ed.), *Contesting the boundaries of liberal and professional education: The Syracuse experiment* (pp. 130-139). Syracuse, NY: Syracuse University Press.

Newman, J. H. (1976). *The idea of a university defined and illustrated*. Oxford, England: Clarendon Press.

Pelikan, J. (1992). *The idea of the university — A reexamination*. New Haven, CT: Yale University Press.

Siedentop, D. (1990). Undergraduate teacher preparation. In *Academy Papers* (Vol. 23, pp. 28-34). Champaign, IL: Human Kinetics.

Smith, J. C. (1986). A response to the Holmes Group proposal. *Journal of Teacher Education, 37*, 52-56.

Thomas, J. R. (1990). The body of knowledge: A common core. In *Academy Papers* (Vol. 23, pp. 5-12). Champaign, IL: Human Kinetics.

Von Vorys, B. (Ed.). (1990). *Peterson's guide to graduate programs in business, education, health and law*. Princeton, NJ: Peterson's Guides.

# SUGGESTED READING

Adler, M. J. (1988). *Reforming Education: The Opening of the American Mind.* New York: Macmillan.

Apple, M. W. (1985). *Education and Power.* Boston: Ark Paperbacks.

Apple, M. W. (1990). *Ideology and Curriculum* (2nd ed.). New York: Routledge Press.

Benthall, J., & Polhemus, T. (Eds.) (1975). *The Body as a Medium of Expression.* New York: E. P. Dutton.

Bok, D. (1982). *Beyond the Ivory Tower: Social Responsibilities of the Modern University.* Cambridge, MA: Harvard University Press.

Bok, D. (1986). *Higher Learning.* Cambridge, MA: Harvard University Press.

Boyer, E. L. (1987). *College: The Undergraduate Experience in America.* New York: Harper and Row.

Boyer, E. L. (1990). *Scholarship Reconsidered: Priorities of the Professionals.* Princeton, NJ: Princeton University Press.

Brooke, J. D., & Whiting, H. T. A. (Eds.). (1973). *Human Movement: A Field of Study.* London: Henry Kimpton.

Brubacher, J. S., & Rudy, W. (1976). *Higher Education in Transition.* New York: Harper and Row.

Carnegie Council on Adolescent Development. (1989). *Turning Points: Preparing American Youth for the 21st Century.* New York: Carnegie Corporation.

Cheit, E. F. (1975). *The Useful Arts and the Liberal Tradition.* New York: McGraw-Hill.

Chu, D., Segrave, J. D., & Becker, B. (Eds.) (1985). *Sports and Higher Education.* Champaign, IL: Human Kinetics.

Clark, B. R. (1983). *The Higher Education System: Academic Organization in Cross-National Perspective.* Berkeley, CA: University of California Press.

Clark, B. R. (Ed.) (1987). *The Academic Profession: National Disciplinary and Institutional Settings.* Berkeley: University of California Press.

Conant, J. B. (1945). *General Education in a Free Society.* Cambridge, MA: Harvard University Press.

Gamson, Z. F. (Ed.) (1984). *Liberating Education.* San Francisco: Jossey-Bass.

Gardner, H. (1985). *The Mind's New Science: A History of the Cognitive Revolution.* New York: Basic Books.

Giddens, A. (1990). *The Consequences of Modernity.* Stanford, CA: Stanford University Press.

Gleik, J. (1987). *Chaos: Making a New Science.* New York: Viking.

Gutmann, A. (1987). *Democratic Education.* Princeton, NJ: Princeton University Press.

Harvey, D. (1989). *The Condition of Postmodernity.* Oxford: Blackwell.

Hook, S., Kurtz, P., & Todorovich, M. (1975). *The Philosophy of the Curriculum: The Need for General Education.* Buffalo, NY: Prometheus Books.

Jacoby, R. (1987). *The Last Intellectuals: American Culture in the Age of Academe.* New York: Basic Books.

Jewett, A., & Bain, L. (1985). *The Curricular Process in Physical Education.* Dubuque, IA: Wm. C. Brown.

Kimball, B. H. (1986). *Orators and Philosophers: A History of the Idea of Liberal Education.* New York: Teachers College Press.

Kirk, D., & Tinning, R. (Eds.). *Physical Education, Curriculum and Culture: Critical Issues in the Contemporary Crisis.* New York: Falmer Press.

Kleinman, S. (1989). *Sport as Performance: The Athlete as Artist* (Big 10 Leadership Conference Report). Champaign, IL: Human Kinetics.

Levine, A. (1978). *Handbook on Undergraduate Curriculum.* San Francisco: Jossey-Bass.

Lynton, E., & Elmen, S. (1987). *New Priorities for the University.* San Francisco: Jossey-Bass.

Marsh, P. T. (Ed.). (1988). *Contesting the Boundaries of Liberal and Professional Education: The Syracuse Experiment.* Syracuse, NY: Syracuse University Press.

Metheny, E. (1968). *Movement and Meaning.* New York: McGraw-Hill.

Morford, W. R., & Lawson, H. A. (1979). A Liberal Education Through the Study of Human Movement. In W. F. Considine (Ed.), *Alternative professional preparation in physical education* (pp. 32–43). Washington, DC: AAHPERD.

Nicholls, J. G. (1989). *The Competitive Ethos and Democratic Education.* Cambridge, MA: Harvard University Press.

Numbers, R. L. (Ed.). (1980). *The Education of American Physicians.* Berkeley: University of California Press.

Wiltshire, B. (1990). *The Moral Collapse of the University.* Albany, NY: Albany State University of New York Press.

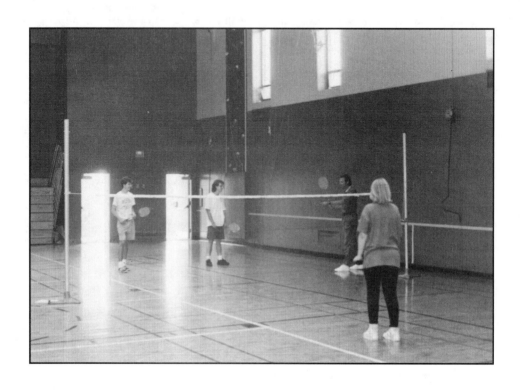

The premise of contemporary kinesiology
is its intellectual foundation:  the knowledge and skills
essential to the study of human movement,
in content areas ranging from
badminton to biomechanics.

# The Premises of Contemporary Kinesiology

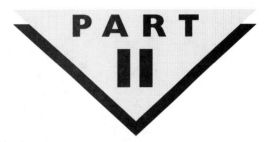

The premise of contemporary kinesiology is its intellectual foundation: the knowledge and skills essential to the study of human movement phenomena. The question underlying this part of the book is how to ensure, through a course of study, that an undergraduate college student may receive a thorough, first-rate education and be prepared specifically to enter a career field in the human movement professions.

A premise of contemporary kinesiology is that exposure to the liberal arts paradigm (described in part 1), constitutes a comprehensive, high-quality education experience that will provide ready access to a range of careers. In chapter 3, the ribs of the kinesiology umbrella, — necessary skill premises for independent learning and for dealing with the challenges of living and working in the 21st century — are delineated in some detail. The other chapters of this section are devoted to examining the knowledge premises of contemporary kinesiology. From the five areas of knowledge discussed in the context of the liberal arts paradigm, a kinesiology student should gain three essential competencies, summarized in the Pyramid of Premises (Figure 3.1) as:

▶ a *philosophic foundation*
▶ understanding of *humans moving* from diverse but complementary perspectives.
▶ knowledge of *human movement* through its scientific bases

Chapter 4 addresses the importance of gaining a philosophical foundation and shows how philosophical knowledge is applied in movement domains. The basic premise of that chapter is that kinesiology undergraduates should be equipped to understand the alternatives in

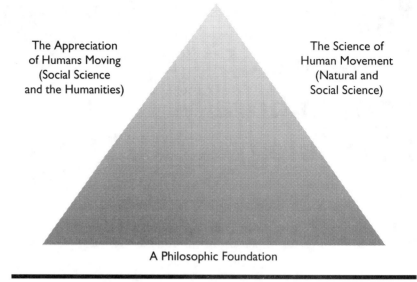

The Appreciation of Humans Moving (Social Science and the Humanities)

The Science of Human Movement (Natural and Social Science)

A Philosophic Foundation

**FIGURE 3.1**
The Pyramid of Premises

a given situation, to select appropriate principles for action, and to make reasoned moral choices. Without these philosophical foundations, options are limited and the quality of life is constrained.

Similarly, thorough understanding of the sciences of the body and its functioning is essential to the human movement professions. The topic of chapter 5 is how natural law and the biological life sciences apply to human movement in kinesiology. Interdisciplinary applications of anatomy, physiology, and biomechanics are related to the broadening scope of the study of human movement phenomena.

The essential premise of kinesiology described in chapter 6 is the appreciation and comprehension of humans moving. This foundational knowledge is approached in three ways in this chapter: (a) as individual and sociocultural behavior (primarily through the social sciences), (b) as a creative process and performing art (primarily through the humanities), and (c) as personal experience (through a broad range of physical participation).

History provides a valuable social context for understanding the evolution of the study of human movement from each perspective. In each chapter, predictions about the future are premised upon retrospective analysis of early development in the field. Similarly, the liberal arts emphasis on an understanding of comparative world cultures is absorbed into the understanding of humans moving by the frequent use of cross-cultural comparisons. The liberal arts goals of incorporating sensitivity to time (history) and space (world cultures) into the undergraduate experience are accommodated by approaches taken to understanding humans moving in contemporary kinesiology.

# Liberal Learning
# Skills

L iberal learning skills prepare college graduates to compete and excel in tomorrow's world. Equipped with these skills, an individual can continue the process of learning beyond the confines of the "ivory tower" of the university. Institutions of higher education intend to create independent learners. A modern university is more than a knowledge factory; it is also an enterprise in the business of acquiring skill. Contemporary kinesiology reaches beyond its traditional focus on acquiring motor skills to embrace the acquisition of each of these liberal learning skills. With its broad-based, cross-disciplinary emphasis on human movement, it is uniquely able to contribute to this larger mission of the university. In each class offered in a kinesiology curriculum, students encounter these skills. The quotient of a skill in a given class varies with the subject matter (for example, philosophy classes stress critical thinking skills, whereas biomechanics classes lean more heavily upon scientific and quantitative modes of inquiry).

*Critical thinking skills* are essential in modern culture to determine the truth of conflicting claims, to selectively sift through mounds of information, and to analytically prioritize competing demands on limited time. Critical thinking is demonstrated:

▶ through an ability to reason deductively (as in the computational interpretation of the mathematics in a biomechanics experiment or the formal logic necessary to reach correct philosophical determinations).

**THE SKILLS
OF KINESIOLOGY**

▶ through an ability to reason inductively (as in the formulation of the general laws of exercise science, informal generalization, and the sound use of statistics).

▶ through sensitivity to typical forms of fallacious reasoning (such as attribution of a causal relationship between two variables in motor behavior where none exists or overreliance on authority when assessing contradictory nutritional claims).

▶ through a willingness to critically evaluate generally accepted understandings (to probe and perhaps to challenge hegemonic practices in athletic institutions, described by George Sage, (1990) in *Power and Ideology in American Sports*, or ethnocentricism in cross-cultural comparisons of sport).

*Communication skills* are a prerequisite for survival and success in contemporary society. Today's information revolution depends not only upon "our collective capacity to assemble and distribute information in easily understood form throughout society (which) will increase to levels we are just beginning to comprehend" (Ellis, 1987, p. 72) but also upon the qualities of clarity and persuasive power that may be packed into a message as succinct as a sound byte. Communication skills may be taught through kinesiology classes that emphasize:

▶ writing clear and effective prose, with subskills of:

　writing informatively.

　writing persuasively.

　following canons of sound reasoning.

　observing the grammatical and stylistic norms prescribed in the *Publication Manual of the American Psychological Association* (generally recognized as the authority style book for kinesiology)

▶ gaining verbal fluency and the powers of persuasion. Debates, oral analyses of articles, and verbal presentations can be integrated into many kinesiology classes to help shift the emphasis in higher education away from its traditional preoccupation with writing ability toward balanced attention to all communication skills.

▶ developing physical literacy — understanding nonverbal communication and using the human body as a tool of expression. Much of the meaning in interpersonal communication is conveyed through body language. (Curiously, even kinesiology, with its focus upon human movement, places little emphasis upon understanding, on controlling and refining meanings conveyed through bodily motion).

▶ improving listening skills. Communication entails more than expressing meaning through written, verbal, and nonverbal language. It also depends upon developing the ability to understand the communication of others. This comprehension may be at a variety of levels, such as literal, figurative, and mythological. Because of its multifaceted curricular focus, kinesiology is a venue for multiple levels of appraisal of meaning. From this critical appraisal, reactions elicited may become the basis of meaningful dialogue.

▶ increasing computer literacy. Computers have become an important medium of communication in this age of technology. The contemporary kinesiology curriculum should offer ample opportunity for students to discover the capabilities of computers for word processing, electronic mail delivery, desk top publishing, and graphic design.

*Inquiry skills* are the basis of independent learning. They help in the formulation of appropriate questions and in the resolution of the answers. Assignments in kinesiology classes may be tailored:

▶ to determine the kind and amount of information needed for an inquiry.

▶ to locate useful information through libraries and other resources.

▶ to demonstrate the ability to apply the principles of historical inquiry, which emphasize verification through critical analysis and comparison of texts and archives.

▶ to develop the computer expertise necessary to identify and use computerized databases.

*Scientific skills* are a basic ingredient of any contemporary kinesiology program. They are essential to success in the exercise science and biomedical professions (described in further detail in chapter 5). A kinesiology graduate should be able:

▶ to demonstrate the ability to differentiate conjectures that are testable by scientific methods and those that are not.

▶ to suggest and develop appropriate experiments or observations.

▶ to apply the principles of experimental design, including:

    a reduction in the number of variables.
    the elimination of uncontrolled variables.
    constructing and testing hypotheses.
    interpreting the data to reach supportable conclusions.

▶ to use the computer to analyze data and in more sophisticated programs to use computerized techniques of simulation to conduct experiments (perhaps in human performance), including those that draw on contemporary research in the total-immersion experience known as *virtual reality*. Virtual reality, a computer use initially developed from air flight cockpit simulation, is highly adaptable to contexts such as the situational simulation of athletic performance and to biomechanical medical therapy.

*Quantitative skills* are the building blocks of kinesiology measurement and evaluation. They include the ability:

▶ to use mathematics to solve problems and support arguments, with subskills of:

    using mathematical concepts in solving problems.
    understanding the concepts of similarity and proportion.
    using graphs and charts to represent numerical data.
    understanding the rudiments of statistical analysis.

▶ to understand arguments of others that are based upon numerical information or elementary statistics.

▶ to use the computer to compile and collate statistics, run mathematically based programs and interpret quantitative data.

*Aesthetic skills*, which sometimes are neglected in formal higher education, are particularly germane to the central foci of kinesiology: the human form and physical performance. A program designed to produce well-rounded college graduates will include learning experiences that foster an appreciation of the artistry in human movement and the opportunity to experience the aesthetic processes of performance. These skills include the ability:

▶ to demonstrate familiarity with the products of artistic traditions that would include not only dance but also aesthetic sports such as gymnastics.

▶ to develop awareness of critical standards as they might apply to these activities.

▶ to understand and experience the creative processes of play and performance.

▶ to instill awareness of ways in which various media forms may develop and reflect aesthetic values.

The application of liberal learning skills and knowledge bases to the study of human movement is the foundation of contemporary kinesiology. These are summarized in Figure 3.2, the Hexagon of Learning Principles.

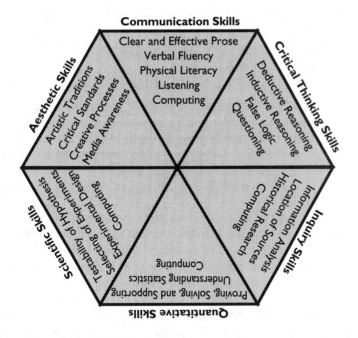

**FIGURE 3.2**
The Hexagon of Learning Principles

The high level of correlation between the knowledge and skills necessary to become liberally educated and those presented in and through kinesiology has implications for university students, for kinesiology departments in higher education, and for the human movement professions.

*For Kinesiology students.* Contemporary kinesiology develops intellectual versatility and flexibility in a variety of ways:

1. The array of approaches to which a student of kinesiology is exposed during a course of study fosters respect for and understanding of various intellectual modes of inquiry and creates a disposition to apply multidisciplinary knowledge and skills to analyze complex issues. This range of ideas and approaches also sensitizes kinesiology students to the need for respect, tolerance, and appreciation of a diversity of perspectives and orientations in their dealings with others.

2. The contemporary kinesiology "umbrella" shelters students from public rancor. Physical education often has met with

disdain. Instead, kinesiology students will be respected if they engage in a challenging course of study that contains a spectrum of inquiry skills that will equip them with the prerequisites for independent learning.

3. Students concentrating in kinesiology will become eminently marketable because of the boom in human movement professions. Students are exposed to an array of liberal arts concepts equivalent to those of any other major on campus. They also are more likely to be accepted for graduate study, further training in professional schools, or employment upon graduation than many of their peers in liberal arts majors across campus.

*For Kinesiology departments.* The contemporary kinesiology umbrella protects university kinesiology departments from the unwelcome attention of "the chief Removal of Academic Waste (RAW) Officer." In a fanciful, but pointedly menacing, dream of the future of physical education entitled *The Subpoena*, John Burt (1987) discussed charges brought against the field by the "RAW Bureau," including violation of the "Code of Academic Usefulness" because "colleges and divisions of HPERD have failed to see far enough to recognize the central issues of the time and to connect with these issues" (p. 155).

Contemporary kinesiology is akin to the "new profession" touted by Luther Gulick in 1890. He maintained that there are "few scientific fields which offer opportunities for the study of problems of greater value to the human race" (p. 59). In the scholarly study of human movement, kinesiologists once again are addressing issues of considerable importance from multidisciplinary perspectives. As Roberta Park (1989) suggested, it is:

*A field of study that draws from subject matter and methods in both the biological and social sciences; however, it also has unique contributions to make. These are to be found in the types of questions it asks and the insights from numerous disciplinary perspectives that it can bring to bear on important issues. (p. 15)*

The issues surrounding human movement that confront our culture are plentiful. For example, Park (1989) identified some salient issues and those who have begun researching them:

*From questions of relationships between physiological fitness and psychological health (Kellner 1985), to symbolic messages encoded in athletic extravaganzas (MacAloon, 1981, 1984), to the cultural contexts that constrain or facilitate engagement in health, exercise and sport activities (cf. Vertinsky, 1987), to the semiotics and hermeneutics of sport and physical education (Harris, 1981, 1983; Park, 1986), a host of unanswered — indeed unformed — questions await our attention." (p. 18)*

Contemporary kinesiologists are asking cutting-edge questions about the human body and humans moving, and they are answering them from multiple research perspectives.

A second concern is that, although the multiplicity of perspectives will benefit scholarship by shedding light on issues from all sides, it simultaneously may weaken the field by rendering it "internally disjunctive." As the indictment of the prosecuting RAW officer would have it:

*In an ill-advised attempt to gain academic respectability you have subdivided HPERD into silly little walled-off compartments, like sport psychology, sport sociology, sport history, sport management, exercise physiology, motor learning, health psychology, health promotion, outdoor recreation, indoor recreation, upstairs recreation, downstairs recreation, modern dance, old dance, and who knows what else. HPERD units are totally ineffective! In no case does the whole exceed the sum of those little compartments, those little pockets of waste. (Burt, 1987, p. 155)*

Contemporary kinesiology avoids the incipient problems of subfield specialization leading to fragmentation into disjunctive units. In the first place, the understanding of human movement is placed in the context of the liberal arts objective of developing the critical and creative intelligence through which men and women realize their human potentialities. This places the research and teaching of subspecialties (which might have become disintegrative if allowed to proceed untrammelled without any unifying guiding principle) at the service of the larger goal of liberal learning. In this way, kinesiology may capitalize upon its multifaceted nature without being internally threatened by it. Departments may be distinguished by being "among the few remaining units (on campus) concerned with whole, integral human beings — biologically, psychologically, socially, culturally, historically" (Park, 1989, p. 18).

The second feature of the liberal arts paradigm of kinesiology that prevents internal disjunction is its curricular balance. The strength of the curriculum is that it draws upon so much that is central to the mission of a liberal education without allowing any subarea to assume paramount importance. No potentially harmful pecking order is established between subfields, and, because of its cross-disciplinary nature, collaborative scholarly initiatives are established appropriately around mutually engaging topics, such as the processes of aging.

*For the human movement professions.* The third and final telling indictment of the office of the Removal of Academic Waste was that, "In violation of the Code of Academic Usefulness, colleges and divisions of HPERD — unlike the useful professional schools, unlike medicine and engineering and journalism and law — you have failed to concentrate your efforts and resources on the development of a high-quality practitioner" (Burt, 1987, p. 156). In total contrast to this alarming scenario, kinesiology does prepare a high quality practitioner:

▶ One with basic intellectual understandings of the body, human movement, and humans moving.

▶ One endowed with liberal learning skills.

▶ One with the versatility to shift successfully within movement professions, empowered to be an independent learner.

▶ One with intellectual values, such as integrity, curiosity, and commitment to continued learning.

▶ One with social and civic values, such as commitment to social and civic responsibility, sensitivity to the importance of the natural environment, and a disposition toward social interactions that will enhance a sense of community.

▶ One knowledgeable about and committed to continuing service in the field of kinesiology.

## SUMMARY

Through a program of contemporary kinesiology, a university student may become thoroughly liberally educated. As part of this process, students will become conversant in critical thinking, communication, inquiry, and scientific, quantitative and aesthetic skills. Because of the obvious benefits accruing from this approach to the study of human movement, (including collegiate credibility, curriculum balance and integration, and enhanced marketability), contemporary kinesiology is gaining acceptance in every type of higher education institution. Liberal learning skills transcend professional purpose. They are valuable, and in many cases, invaluable as ways of learning (in the context of education) and as methods of coping and succeeding (within the context of life).

## REFERENCES

American Psychological Association. (1991). *Publication manual of the American Psychological Association* (3rd ed). Hyattsville, MD: APA.

Burt, J. (1987). Three dreams: The future of H.P.E.R.D. at the cutting edge. In J. Massengale (Ed.), *Trends toward the future in physical education* (pp. 153-157). Champaign, IL: Human Kinetics.

Ellis, M. J. (1987). The business of physical education. In J. Massengale (Ed.), *Trends toward the future in physical education* (pp. 69-84). Champaign, IL: Human Kinetics.

Gulick, L. H. (1890). *Physical education: A new profession*. Proceedings of 5th Annual Meeting of American Association for the Advancement of Physical Education, pp. 59-66.

Harris, J. C. (1981). Hermeneutics, interpretive cultural research, and the study of sports. *Quest, 33,* 72-86.

Harris, J. C. (1983). Broadening horizons: Interpretive cultural research, hermeneutics, and scholarly inquiry in physical education. *Quest, 35*, 82-96.

Kellner, R. (1985). Fitness and psychological health. *Annals of Sports Medicine, 2*, 105-109.

MacAloon, J. J. (1981). *This great symbol: Pierre de Coubertin and the origins of the modern Olympic games*. Chicago: University of Chicago Press.

MacAloon, J. J. (1984). Olympic games and the theory of spectacle in modern societies. In J. J. MacAloon (Ed.), *Rite drama, festival, spectacle: Rehearsals toward a theory of cultural performances* (pp. 241–280). Philadelphia: Institute for the Study of Human Issues.

Park, R. J. (1986). Hermeneutics, semiotics and the 19th century quest for a corporeal self. *Quest, 38*, 33-49.

Park, R. J. (1989). The second 100 years: Or, can physical education become the Renaissance field of the 21st century? *Quest, 41* (1989), 1-27.

Sage, G. H. (1990) *Power and ideology in American sport: a critical perspective*. Champaign, IL: Human Kinetics.

Vertinsky, P. (1987). Exercise, physical capability, and the eternally wounded women in late 19th century North America. *Journal of Sport History, 14*, 7-27.

## SUGGESTED READING

Cicciarella, C. F. (1986). *Microelectronics in the Sport Sciences*. Champaign, IL: Human Kinetics.

Donnelly, J. E. (Ed.) (1987). *Using Microcomputers in Physical Education and the Sport Sciences*. Champaign, IL: Human Kinetics.

Freire, P. (1973). *Education for Critical Consciousness*. New York: Seabury Press.

Giroux, H. A. (1988). *Schooling and the Struggle for Public Life: Critical Pedagogy in the Modern Age*. Minneapolis: University of Minnesota Press.

Prigogine, I., & Stengers, I. (1984). *Order Out of Chaos: Man's New Dialogue with Nature*. New York: Bantam Books.

Safrit, M. J., & Wood, T. M. (Eds.) (1989). *Measurement Concepts in Physical Education and Sport Science*. Champaign, IL: Human Kinetics.

Snyder, C. W., & Abernethy, B. (Eds.) (1992). *The Creative Side of Experimentation*. Champaign, IL: Human Kinetics.

Thomas, J. R., & Nelson, J. K. (1990). *Research Methods in Physical Activity*. Champaign, IL: Human Kinetics.

*"Philosophy is a necessity for a rational being: philosophy is the foundation of science, the organizer of man's mind, the integrator of his knowledge, the programmer of his subconscious, the selector of his values." (Rand, 1982)*

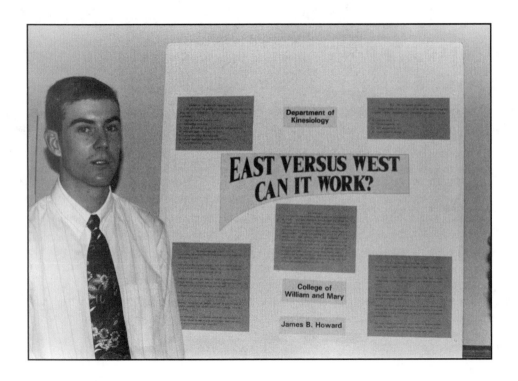

# A Philosophic Foundation

C ultivating reasoned analysis and judgment on matters of enduring concern to human movement is an essential part of contemporary kinesiology. Issues such as purpose, meaning, and value often are put aside in order to get on with other aspects of a particular historical, creative, scientific or technical endeavor. The importance and complexity of these questions, however, justify a central place in the kinesiology curriculum. In this context, courses provide students with a critical analysis of the foundational concepts, theories, assumptions, claims, and limitations of important and influential philosophical thought as it bears on significant human movement concerns. The purpose of this chapter is to:

▶ explain why philosophy is a foundation of contemporary kinesiology programs.

▶ understand the process, structure, and formal content of philosophy.

▶ appreciate how philosophy may apply to each of the domains of movement (previously described as sportive, supportive, and symbolic).

▶ specify ethical dilemmas facing the human movement professions in sportive, supportive, and educative realms and the challenges these pose for professional preparation in kinesiology.

## WHY PHILOSOPHY IN KINESIOLOGY?

Philosophy belongs in every contemporary kinesiology program because it makes sense of the curriculum and provides a foundation of meanings for students entering the field. Philosophy is the glue that can hold kinesiology together during this period of "curricular revolution" (Miller, 1980, p. 216). The very features that impart new vitality to kinesiology threaten its existence. Without philosophical appraisal the explosion of specialized subareas and diversified career opportunities lead to fragmentation and disintegration of the field. Philosophy imparts the breadth of vision necessary to unite and integrate the study of human movement. Overspecialization produces highly trained but badly educated graduates. In the words of a college president, it "has sheltered men and women of broad-ranging imagination behind narrowly drawn disciplinary bounds, thereby discouraging them from becoming educated in the fullest sense of that worthy term" (Freedman, 1982, p. 2).

The skills of philosophy (in particular, critical reasoning and logical and conceptual analysis) are necessary to counter the pinching narrowness of specialization. Used well, philosophic skills make kinesiologists aware of the opportunities of each subspecialty in the context of the overarching framework of human movement study. Reemphasis upon the humanities, especially the philosophic process, is in the best interest of kinesiology. It transforms what might be a narrow, technical, vocational program into a profound educational experience and assures that kinesiology will attain curricular legitimacy and centrality in higher education. Furthermore, it imbues kinesiology students with a holistic vision of the field and an array of personal, intellectual and professional meanings.

## PERSONAL MEANINGS

One of the tragedies of our existence, some have suggested, is the apparent waste of human potential. This can be avoided if students are encouraged to think broadly, to challenge themselves, and to act upon their ideas. Philosophy is a personally enriching experience, one that accepts no "is" without wondering "what might be" and one that does not take refuge in seeking security, safety, or definiteness. It is an intellectual adventure, a process of challenging personal mores and commonly accepted beliefs and of building an integrated system of principles. It is a profoundly practical process. As Ayn Rand (1982) pointed out, "Philosophy is not a senseless parade of abstraction created to fill out the ritual at cocktail parties or in Sunday morning services. It is not a ponderous Continental wail of futility resonating with Oriental overtones" (1982, p. 8).

Philosophy is fundamentally of a useful nature. Philosophy is as intrinsically important to the study of human movement as it is to any other educational endeavor. It gives personal meaning through reflection, assimilation of information, and formulation of ideas and beliefs. The process of becoming is built upon philosophical reflection. The discovery of personal boundaries is premised upon a unique blend of the metaphysical and the physical. Through thoughtful introspection one's essential nature becomes apparent, but only through the test of physical experience can it be validated.

The medium of movement gives kinesiology students a unique opportunity for personal reflection, discovery, and even transcendence. Vertinsky (1991) summarized this latter category of meanings of movement: "This sense of longing for extraordinary experience through health and bodily practices, present as superstitious beliefs and quackery in days gone by, has become in the late 20th century a more subtle phenomenon" aptly termed by Theodore Roszak (1980) a "hunger for wonders," or by some health seekers, athletes, and runners the desire to find the "mystique that borders on the metaphysical" (Kostrubala, 1976), "an escape to the higher self" (Sheehan, 1980, p. 71). Encountering philosophy in the kinesiology curriculum will help students transcend the level of learning "how to do," which is the goal of a narrow technical vocational program. The outcome of this broader liberal approach is that students also will learn "how to be."

## INTELLECTUAL MEANING

To the kinesiology student the intellectual value of philosophy lies in both its process and its content. The process is one of assimilating ideas and formulating principles of action. As Ayn Rand (1982) stated, "Philosophy is a necessity for a rational being: philosophy is the foundation of science, the organizer of man's mind, the integrator of his knowledge, the programmer of his subconscious, the selector of his values" (p. 99). Through the process of philosophy, kinesiology students may be prepared to live a life of self-reflection, to think critically and to act judiciously. Philosophy not only is an intellectual process or something one does but also is content or what one studies. Throughout the ages philosophers have reflected upon human movement. The educated student should be conversant with the ideas that have shaped our belief systems and cultural attitudes toward the human body and its actions.

## PROFESSIONAL MEANING

In tomorrow's world the person who possesses philosophical skills will be eminently marketable. The human movement professions are seeking individuals with long-term resilience in a world of change. Narrow technical skills are necessary for specific jobs, but vocational demands are changing at an escalating pace. Skills that were adequate in one position may become obsolete in the next. Job mobility is a normal expectation. Most people will make career changes during their working life, frequently away from the vocations for which they originally prepared. Useful skills in this market milieu are the liberal skills associated with the humanities, particularly philosophy. In tomorrow's kinesiology marketplace a sense of values, problem-solving skills allowing one to see to the heart of a complex problem, to discern solutions and to weigh their consequences, and a systematic, consistent, and coherent view of life will be preeminent.

The human movement professions, particularly those in the spheres of medicine and education, are overtly seeking graduates with these skills. So important is the skill of critical thinking that a Rockefeller Foundation panel recommended that requirements for teacher certification be based on "a solid liberal education" and exhorted the U.S. Department of Education to "define critical thinking as a basic skill along with reading and writing" (Woodward, 1980, p. 113).

The final outcome of philosophic preparation in contemporary kinesiology is a much needed sense of professionally shared goals and reasoned values. Kretchmar (1990) suggested that, "Many physical educators and exercise scientists lack the professional commitment and passion that could be generated were they only to identify and embrace objective shared values. The general absence of firm value commitments places our profession at risk and may shorten its lifespan" (p. 966). To heed his warning would be to recognize that the role of philosophy in kinesiology reaches beyond the personal enrichment, intellectual viability, and marketability of its practitioners to contribute to the very survival and growth of the field.

## THE PROCESS OF PHILOSOPHY

Selecting a human movement profession is the first of many dilemmas a kinesiology graduate must resolve using philosophical processes. Each individual will be faced with numerable challenges to professional resolve, conflicts of personal happiness and professional duty, and questions of an ethical nature requiring differentiation between right and wrong in a variety of contexts. The skills needed to meet the philosophical demands of an uncertain, changing future should be taught in kinesiology as certainly as the scientific skills needed to understand, describe and prescribe human movement.

In the *Philosophic Process in Physical Education*, Harper, Miller, Park, and Davis (1977) provided a blueprint for acquiring those skills. At the core of the philosophic process is a continuum of proficiency from analysis to synthesis. *Analysis* is a descriptive process involving thinking through an issue, eliminating extraneous variables, and identifying the key elements of a question. *Synthesis* is the prescriptive formulation of a course of action based upon the foregoing analysis. An analogy would be with the coaching process, in which good coaches study the movement patterns of an athlete, isolate key variables, strengths and weaknesses, and factor in the physical potential of the athlete to reach an analysis of the performance of a physical skill. Having analyzed the skill and the performers' rendition of it, these coaches synthesize solutions to performance problems that will enhance the athletes' performance. What coaches do with physical skills philosophic people do with thought processes. This intellectual activity entails analysis of a situation, leading to synthesis of principles of future conduct.

Learning to reflect and analyze before selecting an appropriate course of action is an invaluable lesson within and beyond the arena of kinesiology. This critical approach is essential to resolve commonplace questions such as: Why am I here? Where am I going? How might I get there? The complex of issues that appear in everyday life in and beyond the university requires philosophic skills for their resolution. These typically range from issues of right and wrong, justice, one's duties and responsibilities, the characteristics of a good society, one's rights in the context of those of society, freedom and determinism, the nature of change, and the concept of human happiness, to metaphysical questions of being and nonbeing. Becoming philosophical entails engaging these issues actively through self-distanced, alert reflection. The alternative is taking the path of least resistance that is marked by a certain intellectual passivity. Although this may seem to be a comfortable, nonthreatening avenue through life, it often leads to unforeseen, sometimes calamitous, consequences, confusion, or chaos.

The process of philosophy entails transforming the mind filled with vague thoughts, borrowed undigested opinions, prejudices, unexamined assertions and beliefs, and even some nonsense into one that is perceptive, incisive, and alert. The most philosophic beings seem to have eyes in the back of their heads, much like many superstar athletes, seemingly able to anticipate others' actions and perceive the best course of action almost before a predicament arises. In their detailed analysis of how a student can become more philosophically capable, Harper et al. (1977) suggested that one should:

▶ pinpoint presently held ideas and beliefs and organize them into coherent patterns, often around a central theme.

▶ search for reasoned beliefs by evaluating presuppositions, thinking selectively with an open mind, and developing selective receptivity to differentiate levels of thinking (which may range through hearsay, hunch, guess, fancy, faith, speculation, anybody's unverified opinion, conviction, authoritative opinion, experts' agreement, facts, hypotheses, theories, principles, and laws).

▶ be willing to change beliefs (which entails wishing to improve, being willing to abandon the old to adopt the new, keeping the door of acceptance to new beliefs open long enough to thoroughly test them, understanding the consequences of change, gathering and trying alternatives, and testing the compatibility of selected beliefs with an overall belief system).

▶ change beliefs and develop philosophy using the full range of thinking styles (including mental wondering, intuitive thinking, creative thinking, problem solving, reverie, musing and contemplation, meditation, comprehension of meanings, recall, appreciative enraptured thinking, and rationalization).

▶ avoid problems inherent to this process, both *of condition* (such as overconcern for the practical, seeking security or responding to group pressures to belong, be accepted, be subservient, be content, or be popular), and *of style* (such as overclaiming, making misleading statements, playing up to the audience, posturing, mislabeling, loose thinking, emotional involvement, lack of maturity, a "closed-door" attitude, gullibility, the biased mind, and pedantic verbiage).

▶ eliminate the dangers of arguing at the opinion level instead of discussing at the reflective level, of being blind to false similarity of terms and making mistakes in writing out one's discoveries including:

lack of precision in selecting key words and terms.
lack of clarity in statements of belief.
failing to identify all assumptions.
failing to provide time for scrutiny and editing.
lack of consistency.
undetected contradictions.
faulty reasoning.
lack of organization and systematic presentation.
failing to identify unusual use of words and define abstruse terms.
giving a biased view through overemphasis and indiscrimination.
not being critical in evaluating one's own work.
failing to remove extraneous words and sentences.

Through this philosophical process kinesiology students may be enabled to critically appraise and address the questions that will confront them in their personal and professional lives.

Philosophy is both process and content, a way of clarifying and unifying ideas and a subject matter. Just as the subject matter of kinesiology has been subdivided into units such as history, philosophy, biomechanics, psychology, physiology, and sociology, so philosophy has been subdivided into branches such as metaphysics, epistemology, axiology, and logic. Each area has its own method of pursuing truths, its own form of organization, its own technical language, and its unique contribution to the study of human movement.

*Metaphysics* focuses upon questions of reality. The nature of existence is the ontological (reason for being) domain. *Teleology* deals with the purpose of existence. Metaphysical questions range from the ubiquitous concerns of all humanity (What is the nature of humanity? Do people have free will?) to questions of more particular concern to the kinesiology student (What is the relationship of mind and body? What is the nature of sportsmanship?)

*Epistemology* probes the origin, structure, methods, and validity of knowledge. A typical question in the domain of epistemology is: Where does what we know come from? To answer this query, philosophers study sources of knowledge such as testimony or authority, thinking or reasoning, concrete experiences, intuition or insight, and the senses. Kinesiology provides special insight into what may be known through the kinesthetic sense and the role of physical activity in acquiring self-knowledge. How knowledge is structured is a question underlying educational theory and practice. One challenge facing kinesiology is how to structure learning that takes place through the physical experience so it may contribute to the goals of higher education. The methods through which we acquire knowledge and the relative effectiveness of each are particularly germane to a field of study such as kinesiology, which employs an array of pedagogical styles.

*Axiology*, the theory of values, has particular relevance for kinesiology. Questioning the value of life leads to definitions of personal happiness. Resolution of these definitions has obvious implications for personal goal setting, decision making, and career choice. One form of value is studied through *aesthetics*. Human movement is both a source of aesthetic awareness and a focus of aesthetic appreciation. Using physical performance as the focus of study, standards of beauty and criteria for making aesthetic judgments are established. Aesthetic analysis is a form of examination of the nature and form of beauty in movement, the aesthetic nature of the process, and the artistic product of physical performance. The second axiological approach to value is *ethics*. Ethics is the process of delineating right from wrong, good from bad, moral from immoral, with an emphasis not so much upon "what is" as upon "what ought to be." With the assistance of ideas developed through time by philosophers such as Plato, Hume, Kant, and Mill, kinesiology students can develop principles for ethical problem solving and skills of ethical prescription that promise to be of paramount importance in the complex relativistic context of 21st-century society.

## PHILOSOPHY AND HUMAN MOVEMENT

Philosophy and human movement have a symbiotic relationship in which the branches of philosophy have different emphases in the sportive, supportive, and symbolic spheres of movement. Metaphysical speculation involves stretching one's abilities to reason and to understand beyond the proven and the provable to the domain of informed conjecture (as the term "metaphysics," literally "going beyond physics" suggests). This involves building upon knowledge that can be validated empirically and also upon modes of thought that have gained ascendancy through the ages. Among these, the classic philosophic positions of idealism, realism, pragmatism, and existentialism have emerged to influence western civilization.

## IDEALISM

Idealism, the oldest and probably the most popular of western philosophies, is based on the view that the human mind, its beliefs and its values, is an imperfect replica of the idea of perfect mind and perfect self. There are universal, eternal, and absolute qualities and standards, such as truth, beauty, and good, which human beings may only aspire to but never achieve while in mortal form. Among the protagonists of this position are Socrates (469–399 B.C), Plato (427–347 B.C.), George Berkeley (1685–1753), Immanuel Kant (1724–1804), Georg Wilhelm Friedrich Hegel (1770–1831), Johann Friedrich Herbart (1776–1841), Friedrich Froebel (1782–1852), and more recently in America, Ralph Waldo Emerson (1803–1882), Josiah Royce of Harvard University (1855–1916), and Mary Whiton Calkins at Wellesley College (1863–1930). The value of idealism in today's society is that, through its tenet that the personality has ultimate worth, it encourages a sense of self-worth and an attitude of striving toward perfection. As Harper et al. (1977) suggested:

*The strength of idealism may be said to lie in its respect of man's infinite potential for growth, its stress on emotional and spiritual experiences that transcend the materialistic aspects of life, and its provisions for total personality development — cultivation of powers of the mind as well as development of strong bodies and beautiful souls. (p. 138)*

When compared to idealism, *realism* and the associated philosophies of experimentalism and naturalism seem earthy in contrast. Critics of the ethereal nature of idealism prefer a belief system that accepts only that which can be sensed and proven as reality. Zeigler (1964) succinctly categorized these philosophies:

*Naturalistic belief holds that nature is reliable and dependable. Experimentalism stresses the importance of experience as the only means of discovering whether something is worthwhile. Realism, generally speaking, is the philosophical approach that accepts the world at face value. (p. 113)*

Naturalistic philosophy, a form of realism, is based on the belief that truth and reality may be found in the material things of the universe through science and empirical data. Great thinkers associated with realism include Aristotle (384–322 B.C.), St. Thomas Aquinas (c. 1225–1274), Michel de Montaigne (1533–1592), Francis Bacon (1561-1626), John Amos Comenius (1592–1670), John Milton (1608-1674), John Locke (1632–1704), Jean Jacques Rousseau (1712–1778), Johann Heinrich Pestalozzi (1746–1827), and Herbert Spencer (1820–1903). The idea that binds these and more modern realists together is that a physical world exists independent of the minds of human beings. Harper et al. (1977), summarized the fundamental characteristics of realism as being:

1) *The belief in the reality of matter — the belief that the external world exists as man sees it, independent of any apprehension by human minds;*

2) *the belief that experience is a highly dependable means for coming to know about this external world, and that communication with this external world is achieved through the physical senses;*

3) *the belief that knowledge derived through sense experience is the most reliable (for some realists only) means for man to guide his conduct. (p. 163)*

## PRAGMATISM

Pragmatism, otherwise known as instrumentalism, functionalism, and experimentalism, is regarded as an American philosophy with roots in the British empiricist's movement and early philosophic thought. For the pragmatist, experience is the only reality; that is, we learn by doing. Everything that matters is verifiable through the experimental method (if it works, use it). Prominent pragmatists include Charles S. Pierce (1839–1914), William James (1842-1910), and John Dewey

(1859–1952). Harper et al. (1977) identified the seven tenets of pragmatism as:

1. *experience as the only ultimate reality;*
2. *interactive adjustment;*
3. *ideas and theories as instruments for problem solving;*
4. *the experimental criteria for truth;*
5. *inevitable relativity and change;*
6. *social experiment as a preferred method; and*
7. *the principle of democracy. (p. 184)*

## EXISTENTIALISM

Existentialism is less a complete philosophic system such as idealism and realism than it is a modern "series of statements about the nature of man," which focus "on the analysis of existence, the subjectivity and irrationality of man, and his relationship to the world" (Thomas, 1983, p. 33). In contrast to the experimental method, the existential mode of discovery, known as *phenomenology*, emphasizes logical analysis and insight into human consciousness and self-awareness rather than the tests of experience that pragmatists prefer. Existential thought, which emanated primarily from 20th-century Europe, is associated with Soren Kierkegaard (1813–1955), Friedrick Nietzsche (1844–1900), Martin Heidegger (1899–1976), Karl Jasper (1883–1969), and Jean-Paul Sartre (1905–1985). Sartre (1953) explained the foundational concept of existentialism (that human beings are ends in themselves rather than a means to an end):

*First of all, man exists, turns up, appears on the scene, and, only afterwards, defines himself. . . . Man is nothing but what he makes of himself. Such is the first principle of existentialism. (p. 45). . . . If existence really does precede essence, there is no explaining things away by reference to a fixed and given human nature. In other words, there is no determinism, man is free, man is freedom. (p. 21)*

The fundamental notions of existentialism are that:

1. Human beings must define themselves in the context of their absurd existence. Life is often characterized as being absurd because it is without meaning or purpose. In its extreme form existentialism

seems to be a nihilistic philosophy, evoking feelings of dread, anguish, and anger.

2. People are free to determine their own essence through choice.

3. The premise of those choices should be authenticity and honesty with self and others.

4. With freedom to choose comes responsibility, shouldering the burden of the outcome of one's actions as they impinge upon self and others.

5. With choice comes ambiguity (any situation has numerable possibilities, each with its own potentialities, only one of which may be selected).

## METAPHYSICS AND MOVEMENT

Few ideas are truly new. Our belief systems are generally eclectic composites derived from the wisdom of the ages. Learning to understand personal beliefs in the light of philosophic positions that have prevailed through the centuries is an important part of the process of becoming philosophical. A second goal of philosophy in kinesiology is to learn how to apply philosophic knowledge and skill to resolve human movement issues of imminent personal and professional moment. Preeminent among these are metaphysical issues of embodiment, meaning and purpose, and axiological questions of aesthetic and ethical value. Two metaphysical questions that have direct and profound impact upon human movement and its study are: How do we perceive ourselves as moving beings? What are the purposes and meanings of our participation that are powerful enough to cause us to select physical activity over other choices?

Perhaps the metaphysical question that affects kinesiology most directly and dramatically is the *mind-body* issue (examined in a subarea of kinesiology known as Somatic Studies). The personal attitudes one might have toward physical activity and healthy lifestyles and the societal perspectives on human movement in education are grounded in philosophic notions of the nature and relationship of the mind and body. Idealists, with their emphasis upon the sovereignty of ideas, have tended toward rational dualism. Although he espoused a vigorous, healthy lifestyle, Plato set the tone for the centuries to come in his arguments that perfection and reality are known only by the mind and that the body often serves as an impediment to knowledge.

René Descartes (1596–1650) took the separation of mind and body and the subservience of body to mind to another level through his rational skepticism. He doubted the existence of all that could not be proven through rationality, profoundly distrusted the senses, and subjected all things to doubt, even his own existence ("I think; therefore I am"). This extreme form of dualism (which is often named after its founder) spawned *scholasticism*. Cartesian dualism still pervades 20th-century education as a subtle mandate for the development of rational and intellectual reasoning skills at the expense of physical skills.

The dualistic division into a finite body and an extended mind in a hierarchical order in which the superior mind directs, controls, disciplines, and, in effect, conquers the inferior body has ramifications for sportive, supportive, and symbolic movement. The dualism of work and play, of being studious and athletic, also becomes hierarchical: A modicum of athletic activity may be appropriate to maintain a strong, healthy body (with which to study), but sport had better not interfere with the real business of a university, which is learning! By implication, *sportive* students, blessed with athletic prowess and physique, may be perceived as less adequate students than those who devote inordinate time to study. *Supportive* movement — physical activity undertaken to maintain a body capable of meeting the physical challenges of each day — may be tinged with guilt. The idealist may "work out" only reluctantly, knowing that more important jobs have to be done and that the time spent toning the body could be spent in more productive, work-related activities. *Symbolic*, expressive movement may pose even more problems for a dualist idealist, who would accept the ascetic perception that the body should be controlled. In all probability, reveling in one's physical potentialities through expressive media such as dance would be taboo.

The realist position, with its emphasis upon a tangible, finite reality, acknowledges the importance of the material body. United with pragmatism in a belief in sensory perception and experimental validation, adherents of both philosophies subscribe to the educational philosophy of learning by doing, first attributed to John Locke. The body is a channel for information to the mind and should be trained and kept healthy. A behavioristic tendency emanating from this position is to treat the body as machine and to educate the body as one might produce a performance product (Charles, 1979).

In the *sportive* domain, realists might concentrate solely upon "the treadmill image of sport, centering upon the attainment and development of physical strength, motor skills, and technical efficiency." Morgan and Meier (1988) concluded their critique of this approach by observing that, "In such a mechanistic and often deprecatory environment, the body is restrained, trimmed, trained, and otherwise devivified" (p. 78). In the *supportive* domain of movement, the body is trained, toned, and fueled in accord with the most recent physiological, biomechanical, and nutritional wisdom and is to be suitably mended when it breaks down. *Symbolic* movement, which relies upon creative impulse and treating the body as a source of unabashed pleasure, is at a low premium for the more scientifically oriented realist.

Modern phenomenology presents an alternative perception of the body from the dualistic Cartesian structure. From this perspective a person is a unity rather than a composite of two discrete components. Human movement is inextricable from human being. The body is the primary self, one's way of being in the world, not a vassal, or servant, of the mind or a receptacle and channel for sensations. The distinction is evident in daily dialogue in which a dualist remarks, "I have a body," and the phenomenologist response is, "I am my body." The practical consequences of each philosophical position are illustrated by the different modes of treating a sport injury. Rintala (1991) illustrated how the level of interaction is affected by mind/body philosophy in the following example:

*An athlete has been injured on the court or the field. It's a knee injury. The trainer hurries out to the injured athlete and does an assessment. The injury is a torn meniscus that resulted when the foot, while planted, was hit from the side. To a trainer, biomechanist, or anatomist, if the athlete is simply an object, this is enough evaluation for now. Later time out of action or the need for surgery may need to be determined. But if the trainer and the biomechanist recognize that this is not just a knee but a person's knee and see the athlete's subjective experience, new considerations come into play. To the athlete that is not simply a torn meniscus. 'The injured knee is the athlete's concrete inability to change direction, to put pressure on one's leg, the inability to run' (Thomas & Rintala, 1989, p. 54). It is the athlete's feeling alienated from some part of his or her body. It is the athlete's facing the possibility that a key source of meaning and identity in life may be gone. It is the athlete's feeling isolated from the rest of the team as he or she is being removed from the field. (Rintala, 1991, p. 275)*

Because the body is one's mode of inserting oneself into life, every facet of appearance, health, and well-being has to receive special attention in the supportive movement domain. The healing professions would change many of their practices if the lived body were their dominant philosophy. The concept of body-subject has special meaning in the symbolic domain of movement, in which objective approaches are inadequate and inappropriate to fully comprehend the nature of one's embodied being. The body-subject not only is sensed but also does the sensing. The body is the being. Symbolic movement is not manipulation of an external object but, rather, the physical manifestation of self. A shift toward this phenomenological stance alters the focus of kinesiology from the study of human movement to the study of *humans moving.* The predominant mode of analysis of movement is scientific investigation of the body-object from anatomical, physiological, biomechanical, and psychological perspectives. Recognition that dualistic dichotomies of mind and body are artificial constructs and that "the reality of sport and physical activity is that it is an experiencing activity" (Rintala, 1991,p. 271) has changed the face of kinesiology. Contemporary curricula balance ways of understanding humans moving, which are based on the concepts of the body-object and the body-subject.

This holistic paradigm does not deny the importance of modern movement science. "A shift in focus to include the subjective aspects of experience does not deny the importance of knowledge about and application of the objective aspects" (Rintala, 1991, p. 272). It does replace a Cartesian dualistic emphasis, which served to separate considerations of body from the life of the mind with the nondualist philosophy of embodiment. Implications of this approach run the gamut from a renewed appreciation of personal performance to a recognition that the study of human movement/humans moving is neither separate from, nor less than, any other academic concentration on campus.

Linked to the ontological question of the nature and relationship of the mind and body is the teleological issue of the *purpose of participation.* Underlying this issue is the question: "What meanings do people seek in and from their movement activities?

Because philosophy is not an exact science, answers to the puzzle of purpose necessarily are subjective and speculative. Similarly, the matrix of meanings accruing from an activity change in valency and fluctuate from moment to moment. Even so, it would be a faint-hearted philosopher who was daunted by the improbability of ever reaching an exact, precise, and universally applicable solution to the teleological questions underlying human performance. Recognizing that few aspects of human existence can be reduced to infallible formulae, students of kinesiology nevertheless should proceed to probe those philosophical questions of particular importance to their own selection of physical activity and patterns of participation. While recognizing the pitfalls inherent in dichotomizing any aspect of human behavior, an examination of the meanings typically accruing from symbolic, sportive, and supportive movement may lead to greater self-understanding.

Selecting any form of physical activity is a choice of a medium of personal meaning. That meaning has practical, subjective, and tacit dimensions unique to that individual. The choice is an expression of, and an attempt to identify, personal uniqueness and meaning. Selections of physical activity are based upon the premise of who we think we are and may be designed in light of the promise of whom we would like to be. By choosing one form of physical activity over another and by selecting the physical dimension over other avenues of self-expression, an individual is searching actively for meaning. Eleanor Metheny (1975) cogently summarized the importance of these choices in the search for meaning in life:

*Man's capacity for finding human meanings in his own direct, sensory perception of himself and his universe is the hallmark of his uniqueness as a human, rather than an animal, being. In those meanings he finds the unique significance of his own human endeavors — his own unceasing pursuit of excellence — in a universe filled with infinitely diverse forms of life. (p. 17)*

Thomas (1983) delineated the possible meanings found in the sportive domain of human movement. She suggested that, through sport, one might pursue personal excellence, exert dominance and superiority, define personal limits, take chances, express oneself, and seek altered states and mystical unions (pp. 107–121). Sport, with its clearly defined limits, roles, and rules, provides a setting wherein performance and its improvement are clearly measurable, a controlled environment in which excellence is attainable. Competition provides a medium for mastery, not only of personal performance but also of one's peers. "For some people who play, excellence without superiority lacks meaning and fulfillment" (p. 112).

The other characteristics of sport are contingent upon the expressive, or playlike, quality of the sporting experience. These meanings are found in symbolic forms of movement other than sport, such as dance, art, and sculpture. In his analysis of play behavior, Levy (1978) identified three fundamental characteristics of play:

1. Play is intrinsically motivated.
2. Play entails suspension of "normal" reality and temporary acceptance of an alternative reality.
3. Play involves an internal locus of control.

Intrinsic motivation is "the drive to become involved in an activity originating from within the person or the activity; the reward is generated by the transaction itself" (p. 6). Suspension of reality is defined as "the loss of the 'real self' and the temporary acceptance of an 'illusory self' or 'imaginary self.' Through this form of make-believe, individuals achieve the freedom from the real world (e.g., rules, roles, expectations, etc.) to experience their inner egoless personality" (p. 12). Internal locus of control "refers to the degree to which individuals perceive that they are in control of their actions and outcomes" (p. 15).

To the extent that individuals may adopt the stance of play in the activities they choose, they may define their personal limits. For example, one may elect to don the guise and the gear of a rock climber to master a fear of falling; another might choose to test self-doubts about courage in the face of adversity on the sport field; and a third might seek to overcome inhibitions through involvement in dance performance. Those who thirst for adventure, who seek out vertiginous or potentially life-threatening predicaments may satisfy their appetite for more spice in their life by selecting from a smorgasbord of risk activities ranging from *a*bseilling to *z*iplining.

Another important meaning in movement is that it facilitates self-expression. The physical dimension is a corridor for creativity through which one can channel and explore untapped inner resources. It is also an avenue through which to express unique personal skills, talents and feelings.

Yet another possible meaning, which Thomas (1993) referred to as "altered states and mystical unions," typically occurs when absorption in the play process causes the play behavior and self-consciousness to converge. The resulting experience, during which one becomes immersed in an activity and oblivious to externalities, has been termed variously "flow," "a peak-experience," "oneness," and "the perfect moment." This transcendent potential of the physical experience borders on the religious realm (Sheehan, 1978; Roszak, 1980). Thomas concluded, "Those who achieve flow or mystical union in sport come to know the experience in a unique way, and from all reports, it is significant and meaningful enough to strive to repeat the experience (p. 121).

## AXIOLOGY AND ACTIVITY

Through kinesiology, students will be introduced to the array of theoretical concepts underlying the mechanics of human movement and the machinations of humans moving. In addition to this intellectual study, many will choose to participate in physical activity for the meanings just described. In both the vocational and the avocational senses, students of kinesiology will face an array of choices in the 21st century. A central concern of the philosophy segment of the kinesiology curriculum should be to help students deal with questions of value underlying these choices. These questions may take the aesthetic form (What do I value in this activity?) or present themselves as dilemmas of ethical value (What is the right decision, the morally correct course of action?)

## AESTHETICS

In the realm of kinesiology, aesthetic analysis focuses on the beauty of the body and human movement as it seeks to define what we appreciate in play and sport. The truism that beauty is in the eye of the beholder does not mean that aesthetic appreciation is a function of sight only, or that, because it is a subjective evaluation, it therefore cannot be understood, related to generalizable principles of beauty, and communicated to others. Indeed, the process of becoming liberally educated entails probing beneath the superficial impression, developing skills of critical reflection, refining personal sensibilities, and learning to command language that may convey complex, virtually ineffable, concepts to others.

The beauty in movement is appreciated from the perspectives of both performer and spectator. The performer is internally aware of beauty through kinesthetic senses. The spectator appreciates the coordination, skill, and success of the moving being at a vicarious, visual level. Lowe (1977) categorized these quite different and mutually exclusive forms of aesthetic appreciation in the following way: "The kinesthetic sense of 'action as beauty' can be called the 'subjective aesthetic,' whereas observed pleasing and admired performance can be labeled 'objective aesthetic'" (p. 14). Thomas (1977) analyzed the subjective aesthetic, which she dubbed "the Dionysian perspective" (using Nietzsche's classification), and found it to be "subjective, spontaneous, and somewhat irrational analysis of performance" (p. 73). Conversely, the objective aesthetic, "Appollonian," spectator view is "characterized by cognitive objectivity, criticism, logic, and what is commonly called 'scientific method'" (p.73). Although the performer involved in the lived experience — an inside-out view — appreciates qualities in movement different from those of the spectator — a detached, outside view — both may be able to agree in perspective upon aspects of activity deemed universally beautiful and artistic.

By examining artistic qualities of the human body, its movement patterns, and the powers of creative expression that people demonstrate in and through physical activity, kinesiology students can begin to arrive at an aesthetic consensus. In his cross-disciplinary inquiry into the beauty of sport, Lowe (1977) discussed the body as natural beauty, noting that, although each culture defines beauty in different ways, the physical ideal of the body invariably has stressed natural elegance, the epitome of perfection of natural endowment. Tracing the evolution of the artistic focus upon the human body from the early Greek tradition to contemporary art forms, Lowe identified a continuing preoccupation with proportion, symmetry, and asymmetry.

In studying this artistic tradition, kinesiology students supplement their mechanistic understandings of the body derived from anatomy, physiology, and biomechanics with an awareness of its natural beauty. Likewise, knowledge of how the body functions during exercise augments and enriches study of the aesthetic qualities of athletic performance. Perusal of the works of artists such as Thomas Eakins, George Bellows, Joseph Brown, Winslow Homer, and R. Tait McKenzie reveal the unity, harmony, form, dynamics, flow, gracefulness, rhythm, poise, effort, strength, speed, power, precision, risk, and joy that help define the aesthetic quality of human movement and performance.

## ETHICS

Of all the domains of philosophy, another branch of axiology — ethics — has the most relevancy and urgency for kinesiology students. Ethics impinge upon the conduct and professional practice of sportive, educative, and supportive movement. Kretchmar (1993) summarized the ethical imperative for kinesiology by suggesting that, in a world fixated with productivity, in which material acquisition often is the measure of success, "we must remain sensitive to the difference between what can and what should be done and not allow morally questionable actions to find protection under the umbrellas of strategy and efficiency" (p. 4). Sportive activity is near and dear to many kinesiology students who choose to play sports at levels ranging from the recreational to the intercollegiate levels and who hope to continue to participate in sports for years to come. Some have developed such an affinity for athletic activity that they plan to continue it in an educative profession, such as teaching or coaching.

Modern sport is more than an activity one does without critical thinking. It can better be characterized as ethics in action, a process of posing participants with a series of dilemmas demanding value judgments for their resolution. The manner of their resolution has ramifications beyond the conduct of the activity itself, beyond the public image of sport, and even beyond the teaching and coaching of those activities. As we approach the 21st century, the scenario of the future Miller (1980) envisioned has come to pass. "The time may not be far away when we will judge ethical practices in sport and society in terms of their value for enhancing health and well-being" (p. 7).

Similarly, ethical awareness is vital for kinesiology majors who have career aspirations related to the supportive movement professions (which cater to health, well-being, and the physical demands a given lifestyle may place upon the human body). In the human movement professions that center on supportive movement (ranging from the preventively focused wellness field to curative medical and therapeutic careers), kinesiology graduates must be prepared to make tough choices, even life-and-death decisions, that are premised on ethical precepts.

Specific issues in sportive, educative, and supportive activity seem disconnected at first glance, but often the underlying questions and the ethical decision-making process leading to their resolution have striking similarities. In each case, ethical resolution of complex issues underlies attitudes that shape personal and professional relationships and, ultimately, the course of action selected.

A basic issue raised in *On Liberty*, by John Stuart Mill (1956), which is as critical in the context of modern movement as it was to 19th-century British government, is *the limit of collective authority over the conduct of the individual*. This issue is of concern to kinesiology because professional relationships are based on questions such as: In what ways should the athletic establishment be able to dictate to an athlete, or a teacher impose upon a student, or the medical community control a client? Few contemporary critics would countenance a totalitarian establishment omnipotently coercing the individual to conform.

Conversely, only a radical libertarian would advocate that all the rules regulating modern sport, school systems, and medical practice be jettisoned to create a situation in which the individual rules without limits, indulges idiosyncratic inclinations, and creates chaos out of order. When faced with this issue, human movement professionals must place themselves on the continuum between authoritarianism and unbridled autonomy. Their position is premised upon the issues of rights, duties, paternalism, and informed consent:

1. The balance of power between institution and authority swings on the fulcrum of *rights*. The issue of rights is illustrated by the following questions that are faced frequently in the sportive, educative, and supportive human movement professions:

   ▶ Does an athlete have the right to make lifestyle choices, or do the coach, the educational institution, and the NCAA have the right to coercively enforce certain attitudes and behavior such as appearance (hair length), eating (training table), sleep (curfew), work (study hall, GPA, entry/academic progress/graduation), and habits (tobacco, alcohol, recreational drugs)?

   ▶ Should the athlete or the establishment determine whether and how a student athlete should play (whether to play injured, to foul, or to intentionally harm an opponent)?

   ▶ What rights should students have in a physical education class at school? (What levels of privacy, autonomy, and dignity, and how much control should they have over the selection of transmission of knowledge?)

   ▶ Do those employed in the biomedical, supportive professional domain have the right to make life-and-death decisions on behalf of the patient, or to prescribe profound lifestyle changes, or to withhold treatment?

2. One key to solving the problem of conflicting rights centers on *duties*. If it is determined that an individual has duties as well as rights, the neglect of these duties may provide justification for the exercise of institutional authority. For instance, if an athlete were to refuse to participate in practice, a coach might suspend the player for failing to contribute to the team effort. Underlying this action is the rationale that one should feel an obligation to bear a fair share of the burden of keeping a democratic or collective effort running smoothly. Another, frequently cited duty is that of refraining from injuring others through the commission, or omission, of an act. On this basis, a doctor may be justified in refusing treatment to one who consistently contaminates others with secondhand cigarette smoke, or in physically or chemically restraining a patient who is prone to dangerously violent outbursts.

3. The balance between rights and duties is affected by *paternalism*, the idea that coercive action taken by the coaching staff teacher, doctor, or therapist may be permissible when it is done in the best interests of the individual. Paternalistic action generally runs counter to the principle that individuals should be allowed to make their own decisions, to forge their own pathways through life, and to handle the consequences of their decisions. Paternalism is evident when coaches and athletic trainers coerce athletes into playing against their better judgment or refuse to allow them to make an informed decision to play. Examples of paternalism in the biomedical field are when professionals make treatment decisions on their patients' behalf, or withhold treatment from individuals who persistently continue to harm their own health through lifestyle choices until they see the folly of their ways and adopt a "healthy" lifestyle. Resolution of the questions of paternalism is of paramount importance to those involved in educative movement. Bain (1993) and Kultgen (1988) have suggested that the balance between paternalism and autonomy is important for all professionals but perhaps is most critical for teachers:

*Of all professions, teaching most obviously demands respect for the client's (student's) autonomy. Its whole purpose is to provide the information, skills, principles, and questions necessary for independent existence. . . . The ideal educational system would be designed according to principles that strictly circumscribe legitimate paternalism. Coercion would be minimal, even coercion for the student's own good. (Bain, p. 309)*

4. *Informed consent* empowers the individual in the face of institutional coercion. Simple paternalism, in which a coach pressures an athlete to do something because it is in the athlete's interests to do so,

tends to cast the coach as manipulator, the athlete as victim. In advocating implementation of informed consent, Ravizza and Daruty (1985) suggested that "the coach can compel an athlete when his or her behavior is likely to hurt others, or when it is clear that the athlete does not understand the risks being taken, but not simply because the coach thinks that it is "best" for the athlete to do what is asked" (p. 80). Similarly, the principle of informed consent safeguards the physical education student's interests in school or allows the patient to make an educated decision on treatment. Although it will help to protect the rights of the individual from institutional paternalism, implementing a policy of informed consent is no panacea. As Kroll (1993) suggested, the intention of providing information begs the logistical question of the level and quality of informing necessary for consent to be truly "informed." A further complication is that students may not be able to understand all the information that represents current professional custom (which Rosoff, 1981, defined as the "professional community standard"). An alternative professional premise for human movement professionals is the "reasonable patient standard" (Rosoff, 1981). Through this approach, the information necessary to make an informed decision is selected and presented by professionals based upon their interpretation of their clients' best interests, their need to know, and their ability to understand.

Working through these questions of rights, duties, and informed consent is an important exercise for the relationship of professional and client alike. The ethical issue of paternalism and client autonomy is of more than passing academic interest, for it affects each kinesiology student significantly as the student-athlete-client of today and as the human movement professional and parent of the future.

A related moral question that kinesiology students may have faced already and that will confront them almost certainly at some point in their personal and professional future pivots on issues of *privacy, confidentiality*, and *respect* for the individual. Personal relationships may hinge upon successfully resolving these concerns. For example, a teammate admits in confidence to using steroids to enhance performance, or a fellow student admits, after swearing the listener to secrecy, to cheating on an exercise physiology test, or a colleague discloses in confidence that any violent exertion might trigger a life-threatening heart condition. In each case, the moral dilemma is whether to respect the confidence and privacy of the individual in question or to jeopardize the personal relationship by reporting the confidential information to the appropriate authority.

A similar quandary may face kinesiology students in future professional settings in the spheres of education, sport, and health care. They will have to answer the question of whether they should keep secret the information divulged by students, athletes, clients, and patients, or, on occasion, reveal these confidences to third parties such as families, employers, public-health authorities, or the police.

An allied question is whether professionals, when confronted with requests for candid information, should divulge their expectations to students who probably will fail, athletes who are expected to lose, or patients who may die. Should the professional respect the client's confidentiality, sense of individuality, and privacy and build the bond of trust that may be vital to successfully executing the mutual task (the team victory or the construction of a good learning environment or the implementation of a successful treatment program)? Or, alternatively, might the right course of action be to break the confidence in the name of honesty, or to protect the individual's "best" interest, or to prevent those in the vicinity from being harmed? Does respect for another individual imply both confidentiality and privacy? If so, is intruding into an individual's privacy justifiable in certain circumstances, perhaps to insist upon a urinalysis drug test for an athlete, to probe into a patient's past history without permission, or to search the bag of a high school student suspected of concealing a weapon? The ways in which kinesiology students choose to resolve ethical dilemmas such as these (which hinge upon questions of autonomy and paternalism, privacy and confidentiality) will determine the character of personal and professional relationships now and in the future.

## Conduct of the Activity

Decisions made and actions taken are premised upon an ethical response to a situation. This response might emanate from a relative ethical stance, in which case actions depend upon the situation and reactions are unpredictable. Or, alternatively, the locus of control can be one of the ethical codes established to regulate the primary professions of kinesiology: sport, health care, and education. A question facing all kinesiology students who participate in athletic activity or who hope to teach or coach sports one day is how to reconcile the spirit and the laws of the game, not only at the intellectual moral level but particularly in the heat of fierce competition. Resolution of this issue falls along a continuum from the win-at-all-costs ethic, which essentially justifies any action taken in the pursuit of victory, to establishing sportsmanship as a moral category to govern behavior.

The crux of the question is the viability of *sportsmanship* as a fundamental ethic in the modern milieu of athletic activity. Models of sportsmanship date back to the chivalry of medieval knighthood, the traditions of the English public school, the olympic vision of Baron

DeCoubertin in the 19th century and the formulation of a code by the Sportsmanship Brotherhood in 1926:

---

1. *Keep the rule.*

2. *Keep faith with your comrades.*

3. *Keep yourself fit.*

4. *Keep your temper.*

5. *Keep your play free from brutality.*

6. *Keep pride under in victory.*

7. *Keep stout heart in defeat.*

8. *Keep a sound soul and a clean mind in a healthy body. (p. 60)*

---

Today, ethical codes such as this are incorporated into sport in one or more of the following ways:

▶ in an unwritten form participants tacitly understand.

▶ by inclusion in the laws of the game often under the rubric of "ungentlemanly" conduct.

▶ less frequently, in a comprehensive written format.

For an example, see the *Code*, published by the United States Tennis Association (1978).

Similarly, codes of conduct have been designed to define the norms of standards, principles, and rules in health care fields (such as the Hippocratic Oath [see Edelstein, 1967], the American Medical Association's statement of *Principles of Medical Ethics*, printed in the *American Medical News* in 1980, and the American Nurses Association 1976 *Code for Nurses*) and in education (including the American Association of University Professors 1991 *Statement on Professional Ethics* and the ethical creed for sport and physical educators developed by the National Association of Sport and Physical Education Philosophy Academy in 1993), and the ethical codes of the National Athletic Trainers Association, the American Physical Therapy Association, the American College of Sports Medicine, the North American Society for the Psychology of Sport and Physical Activity, the Association for the Advancement of Applied Sport Psychology. The existence of ideal codes, however, is not sufficient to legislate ethical conduct in either profession, for rule-ethics bring with them a number of potential problems, summarized by Kretchmar (1993):

> *It may not be clear how specific rules apply to unique situations.*

> *Rule books may become so specific that they end up being too large and cumbersome.*

> *Two or more rules may conflict, and it may not be clear which one should take precedence.*

> *Mere compliance with the letter of the law may replace genuine care and concern. (Rules can deflect attention from what may have generated the rules in the first place — sympathy, love, interest in the welfare of others).*

> *Interest in developing and enforcing codes may be a symptom of a deeper problem with ethics in a society or culture. (pp. 7–8)*

Ethical codes, as they relate to daily professional practice and the conduct of research, are a source of guidance, but they require personal philosophical interpretation before they can become functionally operational.

In the realm of professional practice, the personal ethical stance an individual adopts will serve to define the scope and conduct of that activity. For example, under one philosophical premise, professional practice may narrowly focus on winning, personal gain, or material acquisition. Under another, it may be oriented to preserve the status quo. Under a third, the welfare of the individuals involved may be the primary concern. If professional practice is premised upon radical transformation, its desired outcome may be empowerment of the individual, concern for diversity, and social justice. Bain (1993) articulated the latter position as it relates to higher education:

*Ultimately teachers have to deal with the reality that schools and universities vest the teacher with power based on expertise and institutional authority. And they must constantly make ethical judgments about the consequences of their actions in terms of whether the actions respect the dignity and rights of all students and contribute to a fair distribution of cultural, political, and economic resources. Critical theorists argue that the teacher's ethical responsibility goes beyond avoiding discriminatory behavior to include the obligation to empower students, especially those from historically oppressed groups. (p. 75)*

Similarly, health care professionals may base their practice on a variety of principles ranging from turning a profit to providing maximum service to each client, or of providing services on the basis of perceived need, not expressed demand, or of ministering to the ethic of diversity and social justice by providing services to the needy without concern for profit. The ethic adopted will have ramifications for the system, as Edgington (1993) warned: "We will soon experience the clash of two basic American rights: the right to individual choice versus the right to health care" (p. 139).

*Research* is intrinsic to health care and education alike. In both professional realms experimentation on human subjects is loaded with ethical questions relating to what constitutes informed consent, the morality of nontherapeutic research, the rights of children, moral responsibility to a control group, the ethics of deception associated with placebo experimentation, and many others. Likewise, the practice of using animals for the purpose of scientific experimentation raises not only ethical questions but also the ire of animal rights activists, who have devoted more than 63% of the pages and articles in animal rights literature to the use of animals in biomedical research and education (Nicoll & Russell, 1990). On what ethical grounds, they ask, can one justify the pain and death of animals in the interests of the betterment of humanity? The rejoinder voiced by Matt (1993) is that "there is no adequate replacement at this time for animal models in research" (p. 50). Consequently, they must be used in the following five categories:

*Drug testing, such as the development and testing of AIDS drugs; animal models of disease, such as the development of animal models of arthritis, diabetes, iron deficiency, autoimmune dysfunction, and aging; basic research, focused on examining and elucidating mechanisms at a level of definition not possible in human models; education of undergraduate and graduate students in laboratories and lectures, with experience and information gained from the use of animal models; and development of surgical techniques, used extensively in the training of medical students and the testing of new surgical devices and procedures. (Matt, p. 47)*

The final stage of experimentation (reporting and publishing research findings) raises further ethical issues. Safrit (1993) reported that preeminent problems in research include plagiarism, fabrication of data, inaccurate documentation, failure to report discrepant results, citations of fraudulent work, and publication bias. In the high-powered world of medical research, the pressures of scholarly productivity are likely to produce the same types of scientific transgressions as in the "publish or perish" domain of higher education, summarized in approximate order of severity by Roberts (1993), as:

▶ Data fabrication

▶ Data falsification

▶ Plagiarism

▶ Unethical treatment of animal or human subjects

▶ Undisclosed conflicts of interest

- Violation of privileged material
- Irresponsible authorship credit
- Failure to retain primary data
- Inadequate supervision of research products
- Sloppy recording of data
- Data dredging
- Undisclosed repetition of unsatisfactory experiments
- Selective reporting of findings
- Unwillingness to share data or research materials
- Inappropriate or misleading reporting
- Redundant publication
- Fragmentary publication
- Inappropriate citation
- Intentional submission of "sloppy manuscripts." (p. 85)

Kinesiology students are now, and will continue to be, faced with thorny ethical dilemmas as they develop personal and professional relationships and as they conduct their activities in the sportive, supportive, and educative domains. Through philosophy in the kinesiology curriculum, these students may be helped to identify and discuss the issues they will encounter and also to develop ethical strategies for resolving them. For example, in the realm of scientific research, potential courses of action may be weighed against clearly identified religious or ethical principles. Drowatzky (1993) recommended the following common appeals:

- The individual is precious, and the individual's benefit takes precedence over that of society.
- Equality is of the utmost importance, and everyone must be treated equally.
- Fairness is the overriding guide to ethics, and all decisions must be based on fairness.
- The welfare of society takes precedence over that of the individual, and all must be done for the benefit of society.
- Truth, defined as being true, genuine, and conforming to reality, is the basis for all decision making. (p. 29)

By examining these ethical principles, deliberating the consequences of their implementation, and measuring proposed courses of action against these moral yardsticks, decisions may be reached that are "right" and are consistently premised on the same ethical principles. The challenge facing each student is to identify and implement a comfortable ethic, one with which its owner might live in a relatively guiltless, stress-free state, that at the same time gives purpose and meaning to personal and professional conduct.

Kinesiology students should enter the human movement professions of the 21st century equipped with some theoretical tools of analysis, some principles to help resolve the perplexing ethical problems that will face them with increasing frequency in the rapidly advancing spheres of high-performance sport, biomedicine and biotechnology, and the education system. It may be that no one ethical system is entirely adequate for some individuals because of their own conflicting moods and attitudes. Nevertheless, seeking out the most promising options to help chart a course through life seems desirable, however veering that may be. Similarly, the very complexity of ethical dilemmas precludes prescriptive precision. Unlike the more exact scientific approach that underlies exercise prescription or biomechanical analysis, ethics by definition are imprecise and open-ended as this statement by Aristotle (in Nicomachean Ethics) suggested:

## Ethical Resolution in Kinesiology

*Our discussion will be adequate if it has as much clearness as the subject matter admits of, for precision is not to be sought for alike in all discussions, any more than in all the products of the crafts. For it is the mark of an educated man to look for precision in each class of things just so far as the nature of the subject admits; it is evidently equally foolish to accept probable reasoning from a mathematician and to demand from a rhetorician scientific proofs. (p. 936)*

Even given the two caveats that (a) no ethical guide will offer complete universality and (b) total certitude in ethics is an unreasonable expectation, guides to ethical conduct may be developed that are meaningful and give a positive sense of direction. The starting point to this guide should be to steer a middle course between extreme ethical subjectivism (marked by its susceptibility to change [situational ethics], its emotive nature [influenced by feelings], and its lack of grounds for mutual agreement) and ethical objectivism. In its extreme form, the truths reasoned by an ethical objectivist are as incontrovertible as mathematical proofs and as intractable as to make no allowance for cultural relativism (allowing for different customs and beliefs in other countries, in other times, and among different ethnic groups), or for ethical casuistry. *Casuistry*, the study of the application of general moral truths to specific cases, is a problem in athletics, for example, for the objectivist athlete who believes in following the rules and is faced with committing an intentional foul. Similarly, in the research community, how should a researcher who believes in absolute honesty but must deceive a control group by administering a placebo resolve this dilemma? Where subjective positions are too emotional and slippery and subject to reinterpretation on a whim, objective positions can become ethical fundamentalism, which is too inflexible, judgmental, and unsophisticated for the complexities of a rapidly changing multicultural environment.

Having navigated a course between the twin shoals of the extremes of ethical subjectivism and ethical objectivism, the neophyte philosopher may encounter the question of consequence. Put simply, the morality of an act may be justified on the basis of the outcome, or consequence, of actions taken. If it contributes to the summum bonum (greatest good) it was a right act. This is the fundamental position of *utilitarianism*, the most famous consequentialist theory. John Stuart Mill (1962), the originator of utilitarianism, defined the greatest good (summum bonum) as happiness:

*The creed which accepts as the foundation of morals "utility" or the "greatest happiness principle" holds that actions are right in proportion as they tend to promote happiness, wrong as they tend to produce the reverse of happiness. By happiness is intended pleasure, and the absence of pain; by unhappiness, pain and the privation of pleasure. (p. 257)*

The more all-encompassing form, rule-utilitarianism, applies rules of conduct to specific instances, rather like prescribing a particular course of treatment to all victims of a certain disease because it has been found to be most efficacious in most cases. Act-utilitarianists take into account the specific complexities of a given situation and apply a sort of utilitarian calculus to each case to determine how the greatest good can be served through a chosen course of action. While at first glance consequentialist theories of ethics are appealing, because wanting to act to promote the greatest happiness of the greatest number seems quite laudable, implementation of a utilitarian philosophy carries some dangers. One is the possibility of ignoring the best interest of the minority while catering to the greatest happiness of the greatest number. Another is that it might leave open the possibility of doing bad things to achieve good results.

An alternative approach to take in ethical decision making is to base decisions on the rightness of a particular act (ethic of means). Conduct is based not upon the consequence of the act (ethic of ends) but, instead, upon the intrinsic virtue of that course of action. The goodness of an action can be determined in many ways, ranging from evaluating the merit of an action against a particular religious code to deploying a philosophic position similar to that proposed by Immanuel Kant. The Kantian approach is based on a three-part premise:

1. That the act is based on a sense of duty, not personal inclination:

*But beneficence from duty, when no inclination implies it and even when it is opposed by a natural and unconquerable aversion, is practical love, not pathological love; it resides in the will and not in the propensities of feeling, in principles of action and not in tender sympathy; and it alone can be commended. (Kant, 1980, p. 16)*

2. That this sense of duty is informed by ethical law:

*Now as an act from duty wholly excludes the influence of inclination and therewith every object of the will, nothing remains which can determine the will objectively except the law, and nothing subjectively except pure respect for this practical law. This subjective element is the maxim that I ought to follow such a law even if it thwarts all my inclinations. (Kant, p. 17)*

3. That this law is to be followed in every instance: a categorical imperative:

*There is, therefore, only one categorical imperative. It is: Act only according to that maxim by which you can at the same time will that it should become a universal law. (Kant, p. 39)*

Adopting a Kantian ethic would lead to an individual acting consistently according to well established, universally applicable, maxims based not upon the ends or outcome of the act but, rather, upon the means or morality of the process.

The final stage of developing ethical sensitivity entails carefully applying these principles in practice. Care should be taken to consciously engage in ethical reflection, not to rush into applying an ethical position without scrupulously analyzing its strengths and weaknesses. Experimental applications of moral principles in case studies, followed by discussion and review, will help to refine and synthesize an ethical position. This scrutiny will validate the importance of discovering the details of ethically troublesome cases in order to sort out the various valuational variables present in a given context. Once these elements have been determined, the kinesiologist is faced with weighing competing claims and evaluating competing arguments. To assess which claim most contributes to the summum bonum entails measuring each against the concept of highest good that has become preeminent in an individual's hierarchy of values. One approach to measurement is to apply the lessons of history, to seek out precedents that may be instructive to any given modern-day dilemma, to recognize the ethical concepts that have withstood the tests of time. Another is to measure the proposed action against a personal checklist of negative effects that may be as simple as the following. Something is wrong if an action:

▶ *goes against my deepest personal beliefs*
▶ *hurts somebody*
▶ *makes me feel guilty*
▶ *interferes with other people's lives*
▶ *breaks the laws or traditions of my society*
▶ *causes physical or emotional harm to someone; or*
▶ *violates someone's rights. (Thomas, 1993, p. 136)*

## SUMMARY

Philosophy is not remote reflection, far removed from the world of physical activity. Indeed, it provides meaning to our movement and structure to its study. Schools of western thought that have developed through the ages, such as idealism, realism, pragmatism and existentialism provide a lens for the scrutiny of physicality. The ideas of great thinkers serve as signposts to guide our actions. The structure of philosophy suggests ways in which to consider alternative courses of conduct from metaphysical, epistemological and axiological perspectives. Aesthetics facilitates fuller appreciation of the form and function of the human body, and ethics provides a baseline for moral decision-making that is so critical in this day and age.

The onus is upon contemporary kinesiology programs to provide adequate preparation in philosophy so students may be exposed to historical precedents, encouraged to introspectively examine personal beliefs, to develop standards of conduct, to define inappropriate actions, and to apply ethical principles in case study scenarios. The ultimate responsibility of contemporary kinesiology is to prepare each individual to cope with the ethical dilemmas of the future. A philosophic foundation is the premise of principled and purposive decision making. Philosophy extends far beyond the classroom to shape attitudes and behavior in work and play. It certainly extends into the topic of the next chapter: the science of human movement. Every aspect of the scientific process, from the postulation of the hypothesis to the uses of experimental discoveries, is premised upon metaphysical determinations of meanings and purpose, epistemological considerations of the acquisition of knowledge and axiological assumptions about the values of science and the ethical interpretation and uses of research findings. A philosophic foundation is a necessary ingredient of kinesiology, one which will temper and focus the science of human movement.

# REFERENCES

American Association of University Professors. (1981). Statement on professional ethics. *New Directions for Higher Education, 33*, 83-85.

American Medical Association. (1980). Principles of medical ethics. *American Medical News, 9*, August 1, p. 9.

American Nurses Association. (1976). *Code for nurses.*

Aristotle. (1941). *Nicomachean ethics, I*, iii, 4 (J. Weldon, trans.) Buffalo, NY: Prometheus Books.

Bain, L. L. (1993). Ethical issues in teaching. *Quest, 45*(1), 69-77.

Charles, J. M. (1979). Technocentric ideology in physical education: A sociology of knowledge perspective. *Quest, 21*(2), 277-284.

Drowatzky, J. N. (1993). Ethics, codes and behavior. *Quest, 45*, 22-31.

Edelstein, L. (1967). The Hippocratic Oath. In O. Temkins & C. Temkin (Eds.), *Ancient medicine.* Baltimore: Johns Hopkins University Press.

Edgington, (1993). Ethics from the viewpoint of organized agencies: A reaction. *Quest, 45*, 139-141.

Freedman, J. (1982, November). Iowa's covenant with quality. *Spectator.*

Harper, W., D. Miller, R. Park, & E. Davis (1977). *The philosophic process in physical education* (3rd ed.). Philadelphia: Lea and Febiger.

Kant, I. (1980). *Foundations of the metaphysics of morals.* Indianapolis: Bobbs-Merrill.

Kostrubala, T. (1976). *The joy of running.* New York: Pocket Books.

Kretchmar, S. (1990). Values, passion and the expected lifespan of physical education. *Quest, 42*, 95-112.

Kretchmar, S. (1993). Philosophy of ethics. *Quest, 45* (1),4.

Kroll, W. (1993). Ethical issues in human research. *Quest. 45*(1), 36.

Kultgen, J. (1988). *Ethics and professionalism.* Philadelphia: University of Pennsylvania Press.

Levy, J. (1978). *Play behavior.* New York: John Wiley and Sons.

Lowe, B. (1977). *The beauty of sport: A cross-disciplinary inquiry.* Englewood Cliffs, NJ: Prentice Hall.

Matt, K.S. (1993). Ethical issues in animal research. *Quest, 45*, 45-51.

Metheny, E. (1975). *Moving and knowing in sport, dance, and physical education.* New York: Peek Publications.

Mill, J. S. (1956). *On liberty.* New York: Macmillan.

Mill, J. S. (1962). *Utilitarianism and other writings.* New York: Meridian.

Miller, D. (1980). Ethics in sport: Paradoxes, perplexities and a proposal. *Quest, 32*(1), 7.

Miller, D. (1984). Philosophy: Whose business? *Quest, 36*, 26-36.

Morgan, W. J., & K. V. Meier. (1988). *Philosophic inquiry in sport.* Champaign, IL: Human Kinetics.

Nicoll, C., &. Russell, S. M. (1990). Analysis of animal rights literature reveals the underlying motives of the movement: Ammunition for counter offensive by scientists. *Endocrinology, 127*, 985-988.

Rand, A. (1982). *Philosophy: Who needs it?* New York: Bobbs-Merrill.

Ravizza, K., & K. Daruty. (1985). Paternalism and sovereignty in athletics: Limits and justifications of the coach's exercise of authority over the adult athlete. *Journal of the Philosophy of Sport, II.*

Rintala, J. (1991, December). The mind-body revisited. *Quest, 43*(3), 260-279.

Roberts, G. C. (1993). Ethics in professional advising and academic counseling of graduate students. *Quest, 45*, 78-87.

Rosoff, A. J. (1981). *Informed consent: A guide for health care providers.* Rockville, MD: Aspen.

Roszak, T. (1980). On the contemporary hunger for wonders. *Michigan Quarterly Review, 19*, 303-321.

Safrit, M. J. (1993). Oh what a tangled web we weave. *Quest, 45*, 52-61.

Sartre, J. P. (1953). *Being and nothingness: An essay on phenomenological ontology* (H. E. Barnes, trans.). New York: Washington Square Press.

Sheehan, G. (1978). *Running and being: The total experience.* New York: Warner Books.

Sportsmanship Brotherhood. (1926). *Literary Digest, 88,* March 27.

Thomas, C. (1977). Beautiful, just beautiful. In D. Allen & B. Fahey (Eds.), *Being human in sport* (pp. 73-80). Philadelphia: Lea and Febiger.

Thomas, C. (1993). On old wine and new bottles: The transformation of ethical emphasis in higher education, *Quest, 45*(1), 133-138.

Thomas, C. (1983). *Sport in a philosophic context.* Philadelphia: Lea and Febiger.

Thomas, C., & Rintala, J. (1989). Injury as alienation in sport. *Journal of the Philosophy of Sport, 16,* 44-58.

Vertinsky, P. (1991) Science, social science and the "hunger for wonders" in physical education: Moving toward a future healthy society. In *American Academy of Physical Education Papers,* (Vol. 24, pp. 70-88). Champaign, IL: Human Kinetics.

Woodward, K. (1980). The humanities crisis. *Newsweek,* October 13.

Zeigler, E. F. (1964). *Philosophical foundations for physical, health, and recreation education.* Englewood Cliffs, NJ: Prentice Hall.

## SUGGESTED READING

Allen, D. J., & Fahey, B. W. (1977). *Being Human in Sport.* Philadelphia: Lea and Febiger.

Arnold, P. J. (1979). *Meaning in Movement, Sport, and Physical Education.* London: Heinemann.

Bayles, M. D. (1981). *Professional Ethics.* Belmont, CA: Wadsworth.

Beauchamp, T. L., & Waters, L. (Eds.). *Contemporary Issues in Bioethics.* Belmont, CA: Wadsworth Publishing Company.

Burgess, R. G. (Ed.). (1989). The Ethics of Education Research.

Callahan, J. C. (Ed.). (1988). Ethical issues in professional life. New York: Oxford Univesity Press.

Coakley, J. (1990). *Sport in Society: Issues and Controversies* (4th ed.). St. Louis: Mirror/Mosby.

Csikszentmihalyi, M. (1990). *Flow: The Psychology of Optimal Experience.* New York: Harper and Row.

Csikszentmihalyi, M., & Csikszentmihalyi, I. S. (Eds.). (1988). *Optimal Experience.* New York: Cambridge University Press.

Fain, G. S. (Ed.). (1991). *Leisure and Ethics: Reflections on the Philosophy of Leisure.* Reston, VA: American Association for Leisure and Recreation.

Fraleigh, W. P. (1984). *Right Actions in Sport: Ethics for Contestants.* Champaign, IL: Human Kinetics.

Heckler, R. S. (Ed.). (1985). *Aikido and the New Warrior.* Berkeley, CA: North Atlantic Press.

Herrigel, E. (1971) Zen in the Art of Archery. New York: Random House.

Kleinman, S. (Ed.). (1986). *Mind and Body.* Champaign, IL: Human Kinetics.

Martin, H. N. (1884). *The Human Body.* New York: Henry Holt and Co.

McIntosh, P. (1979). *Fair Play.* London: Heinemann.

Mihalich, J. C. (1982). *Sport and Athletics: Philosophy in Action.* Totowa, NJ: Littlefield, Adams and Co.

Osterhoudt, R. G. (1991). *The Philosophy of Sport: An Overview.* Champaign, IL: Stipes Publishing Co.

Postow, B. C. (Ed.). (1983). *Women, Philosophy and Sport: A Collection of New Essays.* Metuchen, NJ: Scarecrow Press.

Purtilo, R. (1993). *Ethical Dimensions in the Health Professions.* Phildelphia: W. B. Saunders.

Simon, R. L. (1991). *Fair Play: Sports, Values and Society.* Boulder, CO: Westview Press.

Vlahos, O. (1979). *Body: The Ultimate Symbol.* New York: J. B. Lippincott Company.

Zeigler, E. P. (1984). *Ethics and Morality in Sport and Physical Education: An Experiential Approach.* Champaign, IL: Stipes Publishing Co.

# A Scientific Understanding of Human Movement

During the past few decades the science of human movement has achieved preeminence in many kinesiology programs. The apparent validity of scientific data and the obvious application and usefulness of many research findings have served to bring courses such as exercise physiology and biomechanics to the forefront. In taking classes such as these, students gain understanding, knowledge, skills, and attitudes about human movement science that represent and embody the goals of liberal education in science. As science and technology in human movement studies become more refined and sophisticated, the tendency is for these areas to become specialized and insulated from the greater enterprise of kinesiology. Yet, all sciences share certain aspects of understanding — common perspectives that transcend disciplinary boundaries. Indeed, many of these fundamental values and aspects are also the province of the humanities and the social sciences. It is the goal of this chapter to:

▶ overview the components that should be an integral part of every student's liberal science education in kinesiology.

▶ Review the emergence, evolution, and contemporary features of exercise physiology and biomechanics.

▶ preview the integrative potential of science in the kinesiology curriculum.

## ESSENTIAL SCIENTIFIC KNOWLEDGE IN KINESIOLOGY

If a student is to be liberally educated and well prepared in kinesiology, certain knowledges are essential. The necessary scientific knowledge is spelled out in the criteria established by the American Association for the Advancement of Science (AAAS) in the publication entitled *The Liberal Art of Science* (1990). These criteria may be satisfied through the study of human movement. First and foremost among these three general criteria is an appreciation of the *nature of scientific understanding*. In addition, the recognition of *integrative concepts* and understanding of the *context of science* are crucial features of the science of kinesiology.

## NATURE OF SCIENTIFIC UNDERSTANDING

The nature of scientific understanding begins with an introduction to *scientific values* and *ways of knowing*. Through the process of probing the properties of movement, students may learn to interrogate nature. This interrogatory dialogue is premised upon a certain scientific mindset. Some of the qualities necessary for this endeavor are curiosity, intellectual honesty, skepticism, tolerance for ambiguity, and openness to new ideas and the sharing of knowledge.

Once the system of scientific inquiry has been activated, the skills of *collection, organization, and classification of information* become indispensable. Among these are careful observation, sound experimental

**FIGURE 5.1**
The Scientific Skills of Kinesiology.

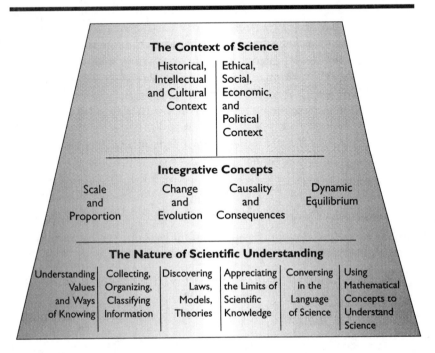

**The Context of Science**

| Historical, Intellectual and Cultural Context | Ethical, Social, Economic, and Political Context |

**Integrative Concepts**

| Scale and Proportion | Change and Evolution | Causality and Consequences | Dynamic Equilibrium |

**The Nature of Scientific Understanding**

| Understanding Values and Ways of Knowing | Collecting, Organizing, Classifying Information | Discovering Laws, Models, Theories | Appreciating the Limits of Scientific Knowledge | Conversing in the Language of Science | Using Mathematical Concepts to Understand Science |

design, the identification of significant variables, and precise, accurate, and reliable measurements. By participating in experiences premised upon the scientific method, students should be afforded the opportunity of *discovering scientific laws, devising models, and developing theories*. This entails constructing and testing hypotheses, challenging the predictive power of theories and models, recognizing the relationship between the concrete and the abstract, and understanding the concept of falsifiability of a scientific explanation.

A liberal education in the science of kinesiology is premised upon not only what may be known through science but also what may not be — that is, *the limits of scientific knowledge*. Any assumption that scientific knowledge is a form of absolute truth should be replaced with the understanding that scientific knowledge is not absolute but, instead, tentative, approximate, and subject to constraints and revision. To reach any level of scientific literacy, students must become familiar with the *vocabulary and terminology of science*. Communication within the scientific community depends upon a common language and shared understandings, both of which should be developed carefully in and through kinesiology classes. Part of this mutually understood language of science is mathematical in nature. The explanatory power of mathematics extends beyond qualification and formalization to the realms of abstraction wherein scientists construct and manipulate mental objects and processes. Students should understand *the role of mathematical concepts in understanding science*, explaining phenomena, and capturing them analytically. In particular, kinesiology students should be able to think logically, make reasonable approximations and estimates, and apply simple statistical procedures.

## INTEGRATIVE CONCEPTS

Certain *integrative concepts* transcend the limits of the boundaries between courses such as exercise physiology and biomechanics. Among these are the sense of *scale and proportion* in the natural world. Through mathematics and analogies students should become aware of the relative proportions of foci of kinesiology inquiry such as human genes, myosin fibers, and blood cells. The concepts of *change and evolution* are theoretical certainties that kinesiology students should come to understand. Without an appreciation of the inevitability of change, students cannot grasp concepts such as position and velocity in physical state and form, in chemical properties and composition, and in biological identity and speciation. The idea of cause and effect is fundamental to science, to kinesiology, and to human existence. In conducting scientific experimentation, students should be reflecting on questions of *causality and consequences*. This entails determining causal relations, seeking explanations and mechanisms for such linkages, but avoiding reaching false cause-and-effect conclusions about the nature of scientific relationships. An understanding of science, and of kinesiology, is incomplete without knowledge of *dynamic equilibrium* and of its application in some specific cases.

## CONTEXT OF SCIENCE

The science of kinesiology cannot stand apart from its *context*. The *historical development and intellectual and cultural contexts of science* help to make sense of the direction scientific research in kinesiology has taken, and thus illuminate contemporary issues. Consideration of the science of kinesiology is incomplete without thoroughly examining its *ethical, social, economic, and political dimensions*. Liberal education must be linked to the real world by exploring the values inherent in science and technology (McKay, Gore, & Kirk, 1990; Whitsen & Macintosh, 1990) by examining the institutions that set directions for science and technology and by stressing the choices scientists, citizens, and governments make about science in human lives. The impact of these institutional choices and policy decisions upon sportive athletic activity and supportive health and wellness-related behavior alike is often global in nature, so the *international context* of science should be included in the kinesiology curriculum.

## THE DEVELOPMENT OF SCIENCES IN KINESIOLOGY

The evolution of scientific understanding in kinesiology has been the primary domain of exercise physiology and biomechanics. (Motor learning and, particularly, motor control also draw heavily from the physical sciences, but, because their dominant thrust traditionally has been motor behavior, with a primary emphasis in the social sciences, they are discussed in chapter 6.) Both are dependent upon understanding human anatomy and human physiology, which may be taught in the kinesiology curriculum or, in some cases, in a biology department. Exercise physiology also draws heavily from biochemistry, and biomechanics employs the principles of physics to analyze human motion.

## EXERCISE PHYSIOLOGY

Exercise physiology is *the study of how the body responds to the stress of exercise*. It is probably the oldest and most well established field of academic study in kinesiology. Certainly it aroused a great deal of interest in the late 19th century when George Fitz, sometimes called "the father of exercise physiology" (Siedentop, 1990, p. 270) instituted the first exercise physiology laboratory at Harvard University. Study in this lab was a prominent feature in the first degreed program in physical education, leading to a Bachelor of Science in Anatomy, Physiology, and Physical Training (Gerber, 1971).

The early research centered on education and health-related comparison of popular forms of gymnastic exercise. A later driving force behind exercise physiology research was the evaluation of the military preparedness and thresholds of tolerance to various forms of physiological stress of the nation's armed forces. Harvard Fatigue Laboratory, under the leadership of eminent research physiologists such as D. B. Dill, continued to play a prominent role in the field throughout the first half of the 20th century.

In the post-World War II period, exercise physiology became the cornerstone of the academic study of human movement in higher education. In 1954, the American College of Sports Medicine (ACSM) was formed to unite scholars in the scientific communities of physical education, sports studies, and medicine. As interest in exercise physiology continued to grow, numerous textbooks were written on the topic, and journals sprang up to facilitate communication within the field. Prominent among these are the *Research Quarterly of Exercise and Sport*, the *American Journal of Sports Medicine, Medicine and Science in Sports and Exercise*, the *International Journal of Sports Medicine*, the *Physician and Sports Medicine*, the *Journal of Human Movement Studies*, and the *Journal of Applied Physiology*.

Traditionally, exercise physiology has been concerned with topics including exercise metabolism, cardiorespiratory support of exercise metabolism, physiologic limitations to physical performance, effects of selected environmental factors on physical performance, ergogenic aids and physical performance, physiologic principles of training, and physiologic effects of training (Adams, 1991). These categories of study embody the nine topics of research emphasis (outlined earlier) by Faulkner and White (1981): substrate utilization during exercise, kinetics of oxygen uptake, anaerobic threshold, efficiency of physical exercise, factors limiting performance, environmental influences on performance, mechanisms of muscular weakness and fatigue, physiological adaptations to conditioning programs, and the role of endurance conditioning in the prevention of and rehabilitation from disease.

## BIOMECHANICS

Biomechanics is firmly entrenched in kinesiology as a popular application of scientific principles to human movement with clearly beneficial applications to modern culture. Biomechanics, a term that combines "biology" and "mechanics," designates *study of the structure and function of biological systems using the methods of mechanics*. To do so, it draws upon the principles and methods of biology (particularly as they relate to the human anatomy and physiology), physics and engineering, mathematics, and computer science.

Modern biomechanics has existed for about three centuries, during which time it has been concerned primarily with the application of mechanical principles to the study of normal and pathological locomotion (Atwater, 1980). During its early, formative years the term "kinesiology" was used to narrowly describe the mechanics of motion, but since the 1970s "biomechanics" has been the preferred title in the United States and internationally: "The few countries using the term [kinesiology] in 1970 have since abandoned it in favor of biomechanics" (Nelson, 1989, p. 7). The definitional specificity of "biomechanics" has led to its almost exclusive use today, which has freed "kinesiology" to become an umbrella term for the study of human movement. Creation of the *Journal of Biomechanics* in 1968 formalized this title selection, as it gave researchers in the field "a focal point for original publications across the entire spectrum of biomechanics" (Roberts & Evans, p. 1). Other journals in which biomechanists publish their articles are *the Research Quarterly of Exercise and Sport*, the *American Journal of Physical Medicine, Ergonomics, Human Factors*, the *Journal of Biomedical Engineering*, the *Journal of Bone and Joint Surgery*, the *Journal of Experimental Biology*, the *Journal of Applied Biomechanics*, and the *American Journal of Physics*.

Biomechanists meet to exchange ideas in various associations. The first International Seminar on Biomechanics was held in 1967 under the auspices of UNESCO. In 1973, the International Society of Biomechanics was founded to promote communication among researchers representing various fields concerned with the biomechanics of human movement (Bates, 1974). The American Society of Biomechanics was founded in 1977 to include the categories of biological sciences, ergonomics and human factors, engineering and applied physics, health sciences, and exercise and sport sciences. Other societies in which biomechanists are active are the American Society of Mechanical Engineers, the American College of Sports Medicine, the International Ergonomics Association, and the Human Factors Society (Atwater, 1991).

The main focus of biomechanics research and teaching within the tradition of physical education has been the enhancement of sportive performance. Application of various principles of physics — motion, force, work and energy, aerodynamics, landing and striking, and hydrodynamics — to the human body in action may provide data on the efficiency of execution of an athletic skill. Cavanaugh and Hinrichs (1981) more clearly articulated the core elements of biomechanics as including the measurement of motion, errors in data collection, kinematic analysis, body segment parameters, kinetic analysis, modeling and simulation, and the analysis of sports equipment. The ability to describe a particular movement pattern accurately has been improved greatly by technological advances in high-speed photography, videography, electromyography, force platforms, and computerization.

High-speed photography is the predominant methodology of *external biomechanics*, which is concerned with the temporal, spatial, and external forces of human movement. Specialized cameras that operate at hundreds of frames per second allow biomechanists to "slow down" the motion so it may be analyzed in minute detail. *Electromyography* is one of the modes of research of *internal biomechanics*, which uses instruments that are generally intrusive in nature to study the activity patterns and intensity levels of muscle tissue. Through electromyography the electrical impulses within muscles may be measured and displayed in representative form such as graphs.

The growth of sport biomechanics is allied closely with advances in computer capability. Computer software allows biomechanists to compare the videotaped and digitized skills of an athlete with precise mathematical models of performance in which the personal physical characteristics of that athlete may be factored into the program. This comparison may isolate and identify technical flaws in the execution of particular skills. In addition to its basis for much movement analysis, mathematical modeling supplies much of the data necessary to design and develop state-of-the-art equipment for athletics. Biomechanics today employs a range of sophisticated measuring gadgetry, which includes not only high-speed cameras and electromyography but also high-speed shuttered video cameras, force transducers including force platforms, accelerometers, and electrogoniometry. Each of these instruments for measuring human performance may be interfaced with computers to create comprehensive, three-dimensional reconstructions of movement patterns. This biomechanical analysis of athletic skill performance, feedback to the athlete and coach, and ultimately correction of flaws in execution leads to better performance.

## THE INTEGRATIVE POTENTIAL OF SCIENCE IN KINESIOLOGY

Scholars in kinesiology widely recognize that scientific research and understanding should transcend traditional boundaries. As George Stelmach (1987) stated in his address to the 1986 Annual Meeting of the American Academy of Physical Education:

*For those working at the cutting edge in physical education and exercise science who are pursuing the frontiers of this knowledge, it is quite evident that the pursuit of understanding is complex and often involves the study of processes, mechanisms, models, and so forth that do not fall within the strict boundaries of a given discipline. The understanding of human behavior or performance requires a multifaceted approach. The plasticity, flexibility, and intricate organization of human performance presents scientists and scholars with a multilayered puzzle of countless pieces and combinations. Thus, the need for interdisciplinary research increases rapidly as we learn more about the cognitive-motor performances in which we are so interested. (p.9)*

This new approach to the science of kinesiology entails:

▶ breaking down the partitions that traditionally have separated scientific fields of inquiry and revisioning the relationship of the world of nature and the study of human movement.

▶ reappraising the focal scope of kinesiological sciences to extend beyond the bounds of sportive movement and incorporate all forms of physical activity.

▶ rethinking the structure of both of the established fields of scientific inquiry in kinesiology — physiology of exercise and biomechanics.

## THE RELATIONSHIP OF THE WORLD OF NATURE AND HUMAN MOVEMENT

The world of nature normally has been studied through the lens of three sciences: biology, chemistry, and physics. Each of these can be adapted to the study of human movement, and they also may work jointly. The knowledge one discipline generates may coalesce with that of another to produce new ways of approaching and understanding human movement. These overlapping modes of study are represented visually in Figure 5.2. In this diagram the triangle of kinesiology is superimposed on biology, chemistry, and physics to show how each discipline contributes to the scientific understanding of human movement. Not shown in this diagram are the interdisciplinary intersections with the social sciences that are creating new fields of study such as neuroanatomy and sociobiology. Because they have less impact on

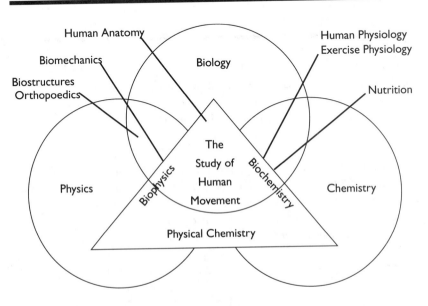

**FIGURE 5.2**
A Schema of Kinesiology Science

kinesiology than the three basic sciences, fields of study that have emerged recently with a focus on the environment also are omitted from Figure 5.2. Although they are not included in the diagram, geological principles and ecological understanding should be included in the curriculum of kinesiology departments that emphasize outdoor recreation. "If we view outdoor recreation as not just play in the outdoors, but recreation that depends on the environment, then recreation can greatly expand and sharpen our view of the natural world" (Atkinson, p. 48).

More knowledge of the relationship of the human organism (biology) and its environment (archaeology, geology and ecology) ultimately will enhance outdoor recreation and environmental awareness (Chase, p. 55). The study of ecology in kinesiology includes topics such as culture, ecology, and social policy; human ecology and cultural ecology; system, ecosystem, and social system; and adaptation, human behavior, and social process.

The combined knowledge and scientific skills of biology, chemistry, and physics with the interdisciplinary understandings of biochemistry (the application of physical methods and theories to the study of chemical systems) form the nucleus of the science of kinesiology. Through *biology*, biochemistry, and biophysics, students of kinesiology study life in all its forms, through analysis of topics such as the cell, energy and enzymes, heredity and genetic material, human development, the physiology of humans, hormones, the cardiovascular system, and nutrition. Through *chemistry*, biochemistry, and physical chemistry, kinesiology students study the chemistry of living systems by concentrating on topics such as energy kinetics, enzymes, the nature of energy, work, chemical structures, proteins, carbohydrates, nucleic acids, and lipids. Through *physics*, biomechanics, and physical chemistry, kinesiology students concentrate on the scientific study of physical law through analysis of topics such as motion, mechanics of movement, force, impact, stress, gravitational forces, energy, work, torque, and engineering. By simultaneously broadening the focus of scholarly attention and integrating various disciplinary approaches, the science of kinesiology is becoming more educationally comprehensive and more generally applicable.

The preeminent focus of science in kinesiology has been sportive activity. Applications of scientific research have been geared toward improving athletic performance, with special emphasis on optimizing the performance of elite athletes. Science and technology are responsible for forward strides in performance enhancement related to training techniques, nutritional habits, injury prevention, skill analysis, and synthesis and fitness levels. Much of this progress, attributable to the

**THE BROADENING FOCUS, SCOPE, AND APPLICATIONS OF THE SCIENCE OF KINESIOLOGY**

research conducted in exercise physiology and biomechanics laboratories, has contributed immeasurably to the public's esteem for these burgeoning fields of study.

While the spotlight of public attention has focused on sporting achievement, with many researchers attracted to the glamour of its glare, the scientific study of supportive physical activity, until recently, has tended to languish in the shadows cast by sport science. The current emphasis on promoting health and quality of life has begun to redress this imbalance in kinesiology. The national debate over health care policies, the National Health Objectives for the Year 2000 process ongoing in the United States, and the World Health Organization's (WHO) policy entitled *Health for All by the Year 2000* are indicators that health promotion is now a national and international priority. Kinesiological research and the study of physical activity are centrally located to contribute to the understanding of health-related fitness. Skill-related fitness for athletic performance has been joined as a major priority within kinesiology by health-related physical fitness for wellness. Position statements by the American College of Sports Medicine (ACSM, 1988) and the American Academy of Physical Education (1987) point to the importance of emphasizing health promotion in the kinesiology curriculum.

Implications for the study of human movement in a kinesiology undergraduate program are that the biological, physical, and chemical sciences are being redirected to include

- ▶ not only extraordinary performance but also ordinary physical activity.
- ▶ not only the physically exceptional but also the physically challenged.
- ▶ not only performance-based research on sport, fitness and training, but also health-related research dealing with the role of exercise in wellness, the prevention of disease, and rehabilitation from illness or injury.

Ramifications for the twin towers of kinesiology science — exercise physiology and biomechanics — are profound as they take on a more expansive role.

## THE CHANGING FACE OF EXERCISE PHYSIOLOGY AND BIOMECHANICS

An expanded scope, multidisciplinary initiatives, and a broader emphasis on the skills of scientific inquiry are changing the traditional orientation of exercise physiology and biomechanics. The insularity of specialized study is being challenged throughout the realms of science. The American Association for the Advancement of Science, which has provided leadership to those involved in science education since it was founded in 1848, recently described and prescribed a trend toward integration and inclusivity in the sciences:

*The move away from excessive fragmentation toward an involvement with the world around, with its emphasis on interdisciplinary research endeavors and interest in problems involving the mutual impact of science and society . . . A shift has taken place toward framing questions that deal with larger issues. . . . Increasing emphasis is being placed on truly interdisciplinary symposia in which science is advanced through the illumination of key topics that will not bend to the attack of a single discipline. Individuals from widely diverse fields — including architecture, law, religion, art, and the humanities — are often essential participants in this difficult and demanding task. (American Association for the Advancement of Science, 1989/90, p. 93)*

Exercise physiology and biomechanics are not immune to this trend. As two eminent exercise physiologists, Wells and Gilman (1991), observed:

*Piecemeal efforts to study human performance no longer attract major funding. Innovative, conceptual approaches that integrate other disciplines and that have wide relevance to various areas of human endeavor are required. (p. 15)*

*Exercise physiology* is uniting with other disciplinary approaches to study topics of concern to kinesiology from holistic perspectives. For example, Wells and Gilman (1991) proposed an ecological model for the study of training for performance:

*The proposed model is human-centered and ecological in nature because it emphasizes the holistic interrelationships between an individual and the biological-psychological-sociological variables that make up that individual's ecosystem. . . . The usual view of training must be expanded to account for, rather than exclude, all aspects of the human ecosystem. A conceptual model of training must recognize the integration of body and mind and the impact of sociocultural factors. Further, it must encompass a lifelong perspective, for optimizing health as well as performance. (p. 16)*

They are joined in their emphasis on discovering more universal modes of inquiry into exercise-related issues that affect the health, welfare, and quality of life of the general population by many leading exercise physiologists who recognize the limitations of specialized and fragmented methods of inquiry. Robert Malina (1991), recognizing that "there is quite often a lack of dialogue between those concerned with the biological or biomedical aspects and those concerned with the behavioral or social aspects of fitness and performance," concluded that "a biocultural approach is essential and provides a broader perspective" (p. 30).

Integration of a variety of disciplinary perspectives is allowing exercise physiologists to collaborate with other researchers in examining topics such as fitness from multidimensional perspectives (Corbin, 1991). Study of the physiological parameters of the human body is broadening to take into account cultural contexts, individual differences, and changes through the lifespan. The multidimensional study of performance parameters is joined in kinesiology by an interdisciplinary biomedical concern for various health issues, identified by representatives of the Institute for Aerobics Research and the Centers for Disease Control as:

▶ *the dose-response relationships between physical activity and variables such as blood lipid profiles, blood pressure, appetite control, insulin sensitivity, and blood clotting mechanisms.*

▶ *the impact of change in physical activity levels on the rates of disease (diabetes mellitus, CHD, cancer) in adults.*

▶ *the association between physical activity and other health behaviors.*

▶ *the association between physical activity and measures of mental health and well-being.*

▶ *the description of specific mechanisms involved in physiologic changes produced by changes in physical activity.*
*(Blair, Kohl, & Powell, 1987, p. 58)*

Related issues of topical interest that engage the mutual focus of exercise physiologists and scholars from allied fields are:

▶ the effects of environmental variables, such as altitude and air quality, upon physical activity and how to recognize, control, and explain the hypothermic reactions of the body to high heat and humidity.

▶ how exercise may affect health and prevent the onset of disease. As medical research controls the bacterial diseases that threatened previous generations, lifestyle choices and pressures are emerging as the primary cause of debilitation and death. The role of exercise in combatting heart disease, cancer, and stress-related disorders, as well as conditions that may be more genetically determined, is being seriously scrutinized in exercise physiology.

▶ effects of exercise on the cardiovascular system, physiological capacities, and the limits of the human body's performance capabilities.

▶ the biochemical causes and effects of exercise relating to topics such as the aging process, obesity, and physical conditioning.

Research in each of these areas is leading to data-collection, information dissemination, and program design of clear benefit to society. Those who suffer from debilitating diseases, such as many heart conditions, some forms of cancer, diabetes, and blood pressure disorders, are

THE PREMISE OF CONTEMPORARY KINESIOLOGY     PART II

being rehabilitated through carefully designed exercise programs. Other people are learning how to prevent the onset of these diseases by maintaining specified fitness levels. Exercise prescription is reaching beyond the alleviation and mitigation of disease to affect the quality of life of individuals of all ages. Because they contain the answers to many of the social and health-related problems facing the United States, the study of exercise physiology and the allied field of nutrition will continue to be the keystone in the kinesiology curriculum in the future.

The application of *biomechanics* to all forms of physical activity and the integration of biomechanics with other disciplinary approaches for a more holistic understanding of human movement are central to biomechanicists today. The traditional emphasis of biomechanics in kinesiology has been performance enhancement in the areas of exercise and sport sciences. Biomechanical studies of sport and exercise skills have expanded beyond the descriptive level to focus on forces affecting movement and on mechanisms controlling force, work, and power output. In this area of sport science, the study of elite performance is being augmented increasingly by the biomechanics of fundamental motor skills performance at all levels of proficiency by people of all ages. The growing awareness within kinesiology that the scope of study stretches beyond sportive movement to encompass supportive and symbolic forms of human movement has awakened considerable interest among biomechanists in kinesiology in three of the other disciplinary categories specified by the American Society of Biomechanics: ergonomics and human factors, engineering and applied physics, and health sciences (Atwater, 1991).

*Ergonomics*, sometimes known as human engineering, is the study of humans at work, whereas human factors consider more broadly the effects of humans interacting and responding to a series of stimuli within a system. Both ergonomics and human factors aim to increase productivity, maximize efficiency, enhance safety, and help humans interact with hardware systems in the workplace. Concern for human movement at work, as well as at play, has prompted biomechanists from kinesiology to study ways in which movement in the workplace may be made more efficient, safe, and rewarding. The mechanical aspects of work stations, equipment, and seating; of load carrying and tasks requiring pushing, pulling, and lifting; of impact forces and accelerations; and of protective and safety equipment — all are factors falling under the purview of the biomechanist interested in supportive movement.

The aspect of engineering and applied physics that focuses on living systems and materials, known as *bioengineering*, is receiving more attention in biomechanics. Tissue biomechanics is a rapidly growing area of investigation that employs the same techniques used to analyze the strength and resistance of the synthetic materials in bridges and buildings to study human tissues such as bones, ligaments, tendons, and cartilage. For example, by thoroughly analyzing the response of the anterior cruciate ligament of the knee to various chronic loading conditions produced by exercise or work demands, biomechanists reach conclusions about the best surgical repair material in time of injury. Similarly, through computerized structural stress analysis, advances have been made in the design of prosthetic devices, of implants in bone that anchor artificial joints, and in fracture fixation devices. Circulatory biomechanics utilizes the principles of fluid dynamics to examine the flow of blood through vessels, heart valves, and heart prostheses, with special emphasis on wave propagation in blood flow, stress-strain relationships in arterial walls, and the deformation of red cells in capillaries.

In the health sciences, biomechanists are studying various forms of supportive movement, surgical techniques, and methods of tissue reconstruction. The contribution of biomechanists with a background in kinesiology has been profound in helping to improve human locomotion in gait labs and in helping the physically disadvantaged to participate more fully in recreational activities through wheelchair design and prosthetic adaptations that allow physically challenged individuals to play basketball, run, or ski more effectively.

Two methods frequently used in biomechanics to analyze human movement from each of these connected but distinct vantage points are profiling and expert systems. *Profiles*, portrayals of the characteristics and abilities of an individual or group, have been used to study aging and disabled populations, as well as athletes of all ages and talent levels in sport-specific kinematic and kinetic pattern profiles. Comparison with baseline profiles compiled through extensive data collection is the basis for assessing normal deviations, responses to environmental and goal manipulations, and skill levels. *Expert systems* are compiled in a data bank and categorized to allow comparison of individual performances with the computer profiles, diagnoses, and prescriptions.

The success of these attempts to profile and predict are premised upon researchers' multidisciplinary collaboration. New biomechanical approaches to understanding human motion similarly are predicated upon recognition of the scope of human movement that falls within the purview of kinesiology and collaboration between scholars from diverse fields, within and beyond the ranks of kinesiology, who may bring their expertise to illuminate a topic of mutual interest. As Cavanagh (1987) reported, contributors to the journal *Medicine and Science in Sports and Exercise* between 1983 and 1985 were in consensus in calling for a multidisciplinary approach. Zernicke (1983) called for a closer alliance between biomechanics and biochemistry in the study of tissue mechanics. Komi (1984) prescribed experimentation involving biomechanical, physiological, and neurophysiological perspectives; and Frederick (1985) referred to biomechanics as an "interdiscipline." Cavanagh concluded, "A theme I would endorse from these three contributors is that the cutting edge lies in the study of problems of human movement in a multidisciplinary manner" (p. 116). Cavanagh proceeded to suggest that primary areas for research and study in the future are:

▶ application of measurement techniques to understanding the movement challenges facing people at both ends of the lifespan and those with certain motor impairments.

▶ refinement of current mathematical models in biomechanics so that research in topics such as optimization might become more accurate in both its descriptive and prescriptive phases.

▶ emphasis upon "the biomechanics of injury — both etiology and treatment — a deeper understanding of the concepts of energy storage and energy, transfer, and a solution to the problem of efficiency of movement" (p. 118).

As a result of advances in methodology and instrumentation and growing recognition of the challenges of new, multidisciplinary frontiers of research, biomechanics classes in kinesiology programs are becoming increasingly sophisticated. As Cavanagh (1987) commented, "A state-of-the-art course in biomechanics today bears little resemblance to the typical kinesiology course of a decade ago. The content, instrumentation, and manner of teaching the course have all changed — and changed in ways that most former students would heartily endorse" (p. 115). Change is perhaps the one constant in the future of the rapidly evolving field of biomechanics. Some of the more futuristic, multidimensional approaches to biomechanics are:

▶ *control biomechanics*, a synthesis of biomechanics and neuromuscular physiology, devoted to understanding the mechanisms that generate and control movement and that prevent and allow recovery from injury.

▶ *ecological biomechanics*, a synthesis of biomechanics and psychology that takes an energy approach to human movement in which motion is considered to be nonconservative and noncontinuous.

▶ *Synergistic biomechanics*, a synthesis of biomechanics and arts based upon the notion that the human movement of a living being cannot be reduced entirely to mechanistic levels of understanding.

## SUMMARY

One of the essential ingredients of an education in kinesiology is the scientific understanding of human movement. Part of the process of becoming scientifically literate involves acquiring certain knowledges, identified as appreciation of the nature of scientific understanding, recognition of certain integrative concepts, and understanding of the context of science. The liberal art of kinesiology science involves activating each of these knowledges throughout the spectrum of scientific perspectives that may be applied to human movement. These range through the overlapping disciplines identified in the diagram of the triangle of kinesiology sciences.

The two approaches identified most clearly with kinesiology are biomechanics and exercise physiology (in conjunction with its allied field of nutrition). Each of these prongs has been expanded dramatically by reconceptualizing the focus of kinesiology. A major emphasis on sportive activity has been supplemented by concern for supportive and symbolic movement. A second, no less influential, factor in the recent evolution of both fields has been a willingness to escape the insularity of purpose and fragmentation of knowledge associated with specialized research, confined by the boundaries of one methodological approach. Collaboration among scholars from various academic backgrounds has produced multidimensional analysis of movement-related issues of concern not limited to kinesiology but expanded to society as a whole.

## REFERENCES

Adams, W. C. (1991). *Foundations of physical education, exercise and sport sciences*. Philadelphia: Lea and Febiger.

American Academy of Physical Education. (1987). Resolution on youth fitness. *AAPE News, 8*, 1-2.

American Association for the Advancement of Science. (1989/90). *Handbook*. Washington, DC.

American Association for the Advancement of Science. (1990). *The liberal art of science*. Washington, DC.

American College of Sports Medicine. (1988). Physical fitness and youth. *Medicine and Science in Sports and Exercise, 20*, 422-423.

Atkinson, G. (1990, April). Outdoor recreation's contribution to environmental attitudes. *Journal of Physical Education, Recreation and Dance*, pp. 46-48.

Atwater, A. E. (1980). Kinesiology/biomechanics: Perspectives and trends. *Research Quarterly for Exercise and Sport, 51*(1), 193-218.

Atwater, A. E. (1991). Biomechanics: An interdisciplinary science. In *American Academy of Physical Education Papers*, (Vol. 24, pp. 5-14). Champaign, IL: Human Kinetics.

Bates, B. T. (1974). The fourth international seminar on biomechanics. *Journal of Health, Physical Education and Recreation, 45*(2), 60-70.

Blair, S. N., Kohl, H. W., & Powell, K. E. (1987). Physical activity, physical fitness, exercise and the public's health. In *American Academy of Physical Education Papers* (Vol. 20, pp. 53-69). Champaign, IL: Human Kinetics.

Cavanagh, P. R. (1987). The cutting edge in biomechanics. In *American Academy of Physical Education Papers*. (Vol. 20, pp. 115-119). Champaign, IL: Human Kinetics.

Cavanagh, P. R. & Hinrichs, R. N. (1981). Biomechanics of sport: The state of the art. In G. A. Brooks (Ed.), *Perspectives on the academic discipline of physical education* (pp. 137-158). Champaign, IL: Human Kinetics.

Chase, C. (1990, April). Cognition, ethics and direct experience — ingredients for leisure in the natural environment. *Journal of Physical Education, Recreation and Dance,* pp. 55-56.

Corbin, C. B. (1991, December). A multidimensional hierarchical model of physical fitness: A basis for integration and collaboration. *Quest, 43*(3), 296-306.

Faulkner, J. A., & White, T. P. (1981). Current and future topics in exercise physiology. In G. A. Brooks (Ed.), *Perspectives on the academic discipline of physical education* (pp. 75-96). Champaign, IL: Human Kinetics.

Frederick, E. C. (1985). Synthesis, experimentation, and the biomechanics of economical movement. *Medicine and Science in Sports and Exercise, 17*(1) 44-47.

Gerber, E. (1971). *Innovators and institutions in physical education.* Philadelphia: Lea and Febiger.

Komi, P. V. (1984). Biomechanics and neuromuscular performance. *Medicine and Science in Sports and Exercise, 16*(10), 26-28.

Malina, R. M. (1991). Fitness and performance: Adult health and the culture of youth. In *American Academy of Physical Education Papers* (Vol. 24, pp. 30-38). Champaign, IL: Human Kinetics.

McKay, J., Gore, J. M., & Kirk, D. (1990). Beyond the limits of technocratic physical education. *Quest, 42*(1), 52-76.

Nelson, R. C. (1989). Biomechanics for better performance and protection from injury. In J. S. Skinner, C. B. Corbin, D. M. Landers, P. E. Martin, & C. L. Wells (Eds.), *Future directions in exercise and sports science research* (pp. 5-12). Champaign, IL: Human Kinetics.

Roberts, V. L., & Evans, F. G. (1968). Editorial. *Journal of Biomechanics, 1,* 1.

Siedentop, D. (1990). *Introduction to physical education, fitness, and sport.* Mountain View, CA: Mayfield Publishing.

Stelmach, G. E. (1987). The cutting edge of research in physical education and exercise science: The search for understanding. In *American Academy of Physical Education Papers* (Vol. 20, pp. 8-25). Champaign, IL: Human Kinetics.

Wells, C. L., & Gilman, M. (1991). An ecological approach to training. In *American Academy of Physical Education Papers* (Vol. 24, pp. 15-29). Champaign, IL: Human Kinetics.

Whitson, D. J., & Macintosh, D. (1990, April). The scientization of physical education: Discourses of performance. *Quest, 42*(1), 40-51.

Zernicke, R. F. (1983). Biomechanical and biochemical synthesis. *Medicine and Science in Sports and Exercise, 15*(1), 6-8.

# SUGGESTED READING

Bloomfield, J., Fricker, P. A., & Fitch, K. D. (Eds.). (1992). *Textbook of Science and Medicine in Sport.* Champaign, IL: Human Kinetics.

Borer, K. T., Edington, D. W., & White, T. P. (1983). *Frontiers of Exercise Biology.* Champaign, IL: Human Kinetics.

Bouchard, C. (1986). *Sport and Human Genetics.* Champaign, IL: Human Kinetics.

Bouchard, C., McPherson, B. D., & Taylor, A. W. (Eds.). (1992). *Physical Activity Sciences.* Champaign, IL: Human Kinetics.

Bouchard, C., Shephard, R., & Stephens, T. (Eds.). (1993). *Physical Activity, Fitness and Health Consensus Statement.* Champaign, IL: Human Kinetics.

Brooks. G. A., & Fahey, T. D. (1984). *Exercise Physiology: Human Bioenergetics and its Applications.* New York: John Wiley and Sons.

Cavanagh, P. R. (Ed.). *Biomechanics of Distance Running.* Champaign, IL: Human Kinetics.

Clark, E., & Jacyna, L. S. (1987). *Nineteenth Century Origins of Neuroscientific Concepts.* Berkeley: University of California Press.

Clarke, D. H., & Eckert, H. M. (Eds.). (1985). *Limits of Human Performance.* Champaign, IL: Human Kinetics.

Dainty, D. A., & Norman, R. W. (Eds.). (1987). *Standardized Biomechanical Testing in Sport.* Champaign, IL: Human Kinetics.

Dishman, R. K. (Ed.). (1988). *Exercise Adherence: Its Impact on Public Health.* Champaign, IL: Human Kinetics.

Donnelly, J. E. (Eds.). (1990). *Living Anatomy.* Champaign, IL: Human Kinetics.

Drinkwater, S. L. (1984). *Exercise and Health.* Champaign, IL: Human Kinetics.

Eroka, R. M. (1988). *Neuromechanical Basis of Kinesiology.* Champaign, IL: Human Kinetics.

Ghista, D. N. (Ed.). (1982). *Human Body Dynamics — Impact, Occupational and Athletics Aspects.* Oxford: Clarendon Press.

Grabiner, M. D. (1993). *Current Issues in Biomechanics.* Champaign, IL: Human Kinetics.

Green, H. (1986). *Fit for America: Health, Fitness, Sport and American Society.* New York: Pantheon Books.

Hall, S. J. (1991). *Basic Biomechanics.* St. Louis: Mosby-Year Book.

Hay, J. G. (1985). *The Biomechanics of Sports Techniques.* Englewood Cliffs, NJ: Prentice-Hall.

Haywood, K. M. (1993). *Life-span Motor Development.* Champaign, IL: Human Kinetics.

Komi, P. V. (Ed.). (1982). *Exercise and Sport Biology*. Champaign, IL: Human Kinetics.

Kreighbaum, E., & Barthels, K. M. (1990). *Biomechanics: A Qualitative Approach for Studying Human Movement*. New York: Macmillan Publishing Co.

Latash, M. L. (1993). *Control of Human Movement*. Champaign, IL: Human Kinetics.

LeVeau, B. F. (1992). *Williams and Lissner's Biomechanics of Human Motion*. Philadelphia: W. B. Saunders Co.

Malina, R. M., & Bouchard, C. (1991). *Growth, Maturation and Physical Activity*. Champaign, IL: Human Kinetics.

Nazar, K. (Eds.). (1990). *International Perspectives in Exercise Physiology*. Champaign, IL: Human Kinetics.

Newell, K. M., & Corcos, D. M. (1993). *Variability and Motor Control*. Champaign, IL: Human Kinetics.

Nordin, M., & Frankel, V. H. (1989). *Basic Biomechanics of the Musculoskeletal System*. Philadelphia: Lea and Febiger.

Perren, S. (Ed.). (1985). *Biomechanics: Principles and Applications*. Boston: Mastinus Nijhoff.

Pollock, & Wilmare, J. (1990). *Exercise in Health and Disease: Evaluation and Prescription for Prevention and Rehabilitation*. Philadelphia: W. G. Saunders.

Schmidt, R. A. (1991). *Motor Learning and Performance*. Champaign, IL: Human Kinetics.

Schmidt, R. A. (1988). *Motor Control and Learning*. Champaign, IL: Human Kinetics.

Shurkin, J. (1985). *Engines of the Mind*. New York: Washington Square Press.

Skinner, J. S., Corbin, C. B., Landers, D. M., Mastin, P. E. & Wells, C. L. (Eds.). (1989). *Future Directions in Exercise and Sport Science Research*. Champaign, IL: Human Kinetics.

Smith, E. L. & Serfass, R. C. (Eds.). (1981). *Exercise and Aging: The Scientific Basis*. Hillside, NJ: Enslow.

Snyder, C. W., & Abernethy, B. (Eds.). (1992). *The Creative Side of Experimentation*. Champaign, IL: Human Kinetics.

Sutton, J. R., & Brock, R. M. (Eds.). (1986). *Sports Medicine for the Mature Athlete*. Indianapolis: Benchmark Press.

Tortora, G. J., & Grabowski, S. R. (Eds.). (1993). *Principles of Anatomy and Physiology*. New York: HarperCollins College Publishers.

Vaughan, C. L., Davis, B. L., & O'Connor, J. *Gait Analysis Laboratory*. Champaign, IL: Human Kinetics.

Vaughan, C. L., Besser, M. P., Sussman, M. D., & Bowshes, K. A. (Eds.). (1992). *Biomechanics of Human Gait*. Champaign, IL: Human Kinetics.

Wells, C. L. (1985). *Women, Sport and Performance: A Physiological Perspective*. Champaign, IL: Human Kinetics.

Willis, J. D., & Campbell, L. F. (1992). *Exercise Psychology*. Champaign, IL: Human Kinetics.

Winter, D. A. (1979). *Biomechanics of Human Movement*. Toronto: John Wiley and Sons.

*"Examining expressive, performative meanings of sport*
*requires more alteration to humanistic frameworks. . . . Investigation*
*of underlying social structures requires attention*
*to social science frameworks."* (Harris, 1989)

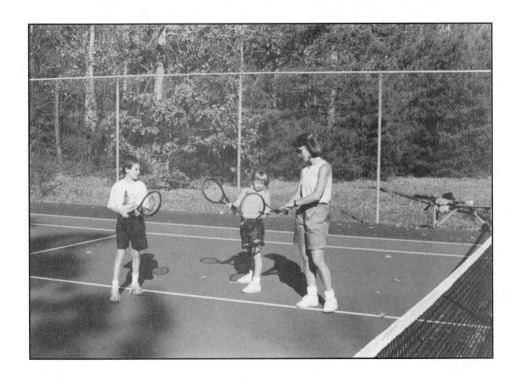

*"Kinesiology without participation in movement activities*
*is like a music program in which no one ever plays an instrument."*
(Bain, 1991)

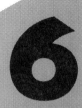

# The Holistic Understanding of Humans Moving

Without a philosophic foundation in the curriculum (chapter 4), a kinesiology department would be casting out its graduates into society to drift aimlessly, leaving them vulnerable to the currents of change, lacking purpose or principle. Without providing a thorough grounding in the biological and physical sciences as they relate to human movement (chapter 5), kinesiology departments would be remiss, for their students would not understand the functioning of the body in motion. Without being made aware of the human dimensions of physical activity, students would emerge from their kinesiology concentration with a mechanistic, technical understanding of how the body works but with no comprehension of the human factors. Students would have completed a course of study in human movement without understanding humans moving.

The humanities and social sciences have complementary functions in studying humans moving. Janet Harris (1989), a leading social scientist in sports studies, broached the question of how social science and the humanities are linked to sport:

*Examining expressive, performative meanings of sport requires more attention to humanistic frameworks, especially some of those that combine ideas from symbolic anthropology, theater and film studies, literary studies, and communication studies. Investigation of underlying social structures requires attention to social science frameworks, especially those in sociology, anthropology, and political science. History provides a useful diachronic social context for both levels. (p. 344)*

Similar collaborative, cross-disciplinary scholarship is extended beyond the realm of sport to encompass every dimension of humans moving in kinesiology. The social sciences have a primary role in examining aspects of the movement process as individual behavior and sociocultural interaction. Approaches from the humanities are especially useful in illuminating the expressive, performative features of human activity. In addition, to truly appreciate the qualities of physical activity, students of kinesiology step beyond the study of its cognitive features to personally experience it in its many forms. Through the combined knowledge of the social sciences, the humanities, and personal experience, a kinesiology student comes to appreciate and comprehend humans moving.

## EXAMINING HUMAN MOVEMENT BEHAVIOR THROUGH THE SOCIAL SCIENCES

Human movement is a fundamental form of individual and sociocultural behavior. At the psychological level it is no less than the physical manifestation of the personal psyche, the visible interaction of mind with body (see chapter 4 for further discussion of embodiment from the philosophic perspective). The relationship between physical activity and sociocultural behavior is no less profound. Through various forms of movement, people interact socially, develop group relationships and are exposed to the processes and institutions of their society and other cultures.

The most visible form of movement in many societies is sport. It has become so pervasive in this culture that it is a primary socializing agent for many, a cultural institution of some magnitude and (given the television viewing habits of the nation) one of the major avenues of anthropological awareness for the general public. Kinesiology, with its concentration on sport and other human movement phenomena, is situated to contribute in unique ways to the goals of a liberal education. It can promote understanding of personal behavior, interpersonal relationships and group dynamics, the institutions of society and global cultures. Study of these facets of human behavior are incorporated into contemporary kinesiology through the *integration* of disciplinary perspectives including psychology, sociology, and anthropology. Psychology deals with the behavior of individual human beings; sociology is concerned with social processes and institutions; and anthropology examines cultural adaptation and, through cross-cultural comparison, the differences between and among world cultures. Where psychology, sociology, and anthropology overlap, the following fields of inquiry have developed: social psychology (which examines individual behavior in the context of social relationships), social anthropology (the cross-cultural study of human social systems), and the area of personality and culture (which involves study of the effect of cultural differences on the individual personality). The social science schema presented in Figure 6.1 indicates that the primary disciplines of psychology, sociology, and anthropology spawned traditional foci within physical education and sport studies in the past. The areas that emerged and flourished during the latter part of the 20th century were sport sociology, sport psychology, and motor development and motor learning. Recently, the willingness to explore and develop academic territory at the frontiers of each discipline, to develop subfields where they overlap, and to subsume the entire venture within a liberal arts paradigm have led to the emergence of contemporary kinesiology social science: a multi-disciplinary approach to the study of the human movement behavior of the individual and society. As a foundation for future learning, let's first take a look back.

**A LOOK BACK**

**Sport Sociology**

Sport sociology arose in response to the growth of modern sport in the latter half of the 20th century. A few scholars from sociology and a greater number of physical educators interested in the sociologic aspects of sport pioneered the sociology of sport. They were hindered in

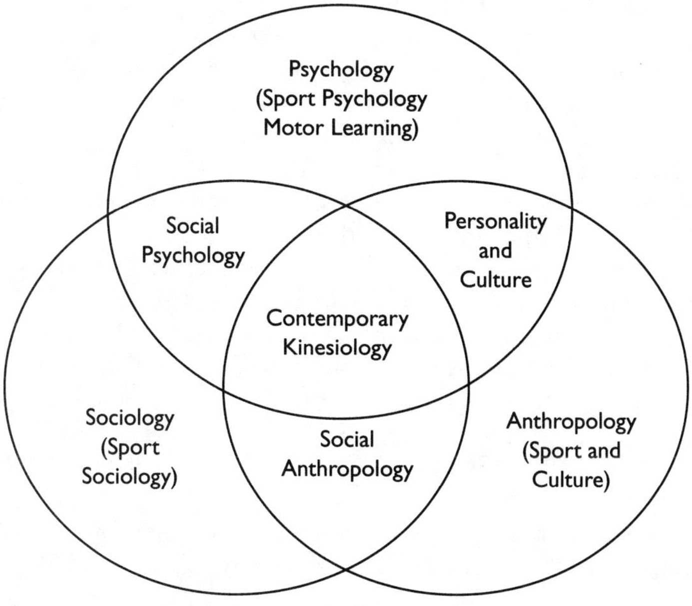

**FIGURE 6.1**
A Social Science Schema

their efforts at first by the misperceptions that sport is a frivolous activity divorced from the real world and that sport emphasizes physical, not social, interaction. As sport became culturally ubiquitous, however, it became apparent that its structure, function, and processes affect human social behavior, and that data necessary for research were readily available that were recorded precisely and publicly. Consequently, sport has become a rewarding site for sociocultural study and research not only in the United States but also, because of its global appeal, it provides invaluable cross-cultural comparisons.

Early pioneers of sport sociology as a subdiscipline were Popplow and Plessner in the early 1950s in Europe, but not until 1965 did Kenyon and Loy (in their article, "Toward a Sociology of Sport") effectively challenge the field to develop the subdiscipline of sport sociology in North America. Since that time, a burgeoning group of scholars has become dedicated to the study of sport and social institutions, social stratification, and socialization. Many are employed in higher education, attend meetings of associations such as the North American Society for the Study of Sport (NASSS), the Sport Sociology Academy of the American Alliance of Health, Physical Education, Recreation and Dance (AAHPERD), and the American Sociological Association, and publish their findings in journals including the *Sociology of Sport Journal*, the *Journal of Sport and Social Issues*, the *Journal of Sport Behavior*, *Quest*, the *Arena Review*, and the *International Review of the Sociology of Sport*.

The uniting force behind the research and teaching of sport sociologists is their desire to understand and, in some cases, to change sport as a social construct. Sport is generally accepted to be a microcosm of society to the extent that it mirrors prevalent social processes, roles and relationships, values, and institutional hierarchy. Approaches and methodologies range from the objective normative approach, which seeks to better understand and predict human behavior through careful observational and statistical analyses of the sport setting, to a form of sociological activism that seeks to go beyond understanding to actually changing perceived inequities in sport. George Sage (1990) characterized the latter position as premised upon the relativistic notion of reality as a social construct, sensitivity to the influence of social structure upon human behavior, and a quality of sociological imagination featuring historical, comparative, and critical awareness. Critical theorists generally accept as their starting premise the principles that sport reflects culture and society, reinforces social inequalities, and is a vehicle for social conflict (McPherson, Curtis, & Loy, 1989) and that it is essentially hegemonic rather than pluralistic (Sage, 1990).

The research tools of sport sociologists are interviews, statistics, library and archival research, questionnaires, surveys, document analysis, direct observation, and controlled experimentation of a socio-metric nature. They use these tools:

▶ to understand sport as a social institution and its linkages with education, religion, politics, economics, and the legal system.

▶ to analyze socialization into and through sport.

▶ to study social stratification issues such as the relationship between sport and social class, social mobility through sport, and equal treatment revolving around gender, race, and age.

## Sport Psychology

The visibility of elite athletics and the accompanying drive to excel have spotlighted not only physiological and biomechanical advances but also how the mind can be harnessed to maximize performance. Phenomenal performances that seemed to transcend and even defy the technological and physiological parameters of the times, such as Bob Beaman's 1968 Olympic long jump, have added credence to claims that psychological territory is the final frontier in performance enhancement. The beginnings of the formal organization of sport psychology can be traced to the Olympic movement. The International Society of Sport Psychology (ISSP) was founded in 1965 to administer the first International Congress of Sport Psychology following the Olympic Games in Rome. The North American Society for the Psychology of Sport and Physical Activity (NASPSPA) was established in 1966 to help organize the second International Congress, which was to be hosted in the United States because of the political and civil unrest in Mexico City.

From these early beginnings emerged the first generation of sport psychologists. They generally held doctorates in physical education and had some academic background in psychology. Building on their interests in sport and the effects on human motor performance of factors such as motivation, arousal, anxiety, and personality theory, they proceeded to develop sport psychology programs in North American universities. In Europe, sport psychology and motor learning were inextricably linked and were invariably housed in departments of psychology. In the United States, however, they developed as two separate and distinct subfields within the emerging academic discipline of physical education. During its recent history the research interest of scholars in sport psychology has shifted from an emphasis upon personality and its interrelationship with performance to an emphasis on the appropriation, testing, and modification of mainstream psychological theory to the purposes of sport. The most recent trend within sport psychology has been away from a clinical form of academic research, which may be informative but not necessarily immediately useful, toward the client-centered application of psychological technique to enhance performance. In 1985, the Association for the Advancement of Applied Sport Psychology and the *Journal of Applied Sport Psychology* were inaugurated to give direction to the applied branch of the field. Clinical and applied psychology alike established channels of communication such as the *International Journal of Psychology of Sport*, the *Journal of Sport and Exercise Psychology*, the *Sport Psychologist*, and the *Journal of Sport Behavior*.

## Motor Development, Motor Learning and Motor Control

Motor development and motor learning emerged from their common parent, psychology. They share a basic heritage of developmental psychology, learning theories, psychometric evaluation techniques, and skill acquisition. *Motor development* is concerned primarily with the interrelationship of physical ability, skill development, and the maturation process. More specifically, motor development is concerned with:

▶ questions of heredity and environment.
▶ the variables of age and sex.
▶ the progression of motor skill development.
▶ perceptual-motor development.
▶ the effects of intelligence upon motor performance.
▶ the quality of cognitive processes during skill acquisition.
▶ physical fitness and children.
▶ youth sports development. (Colfer, Hamilton, Magill, & Hamilton, 1986)

*Motor learning* traditionally has centered on:

▶ acquisition of motor skills.
▶ learning processes.
▶ stages of learning.
▶ variables underlying motor performance.
▶ practice conditions.
▶ knowledge of results.
▶ the role of memory.

The emergence of motor control as a major concern of motor learning has augmented the predominant psychological approach to the study of human motor performance with a neurophysiological emphasis. For more than a decade, motor learning experts, biomechanists, exercise physiologists, and neuroscientists have been working together to explain how patterns of voluntary movement result from interaction between the body and the environment and between different structures of the body. Issues studied in motor control include:

- single and multi-joint movements.
- the emergence of electromyographic patterns.
- the phenomena of motor learning and variability.
- postural control and preprogramming.
- pathological aspects of motor control in disorders such as spasticity, Parkinson's disease, and Down syndrome. (Latash, 1993)

Rather than manipulate environmental variables, such as feedback, to investigate how they might affect task performance, motor control researchers have begun to study underlying cognitive processes and the interaction of the nervous system with the muscular system. Motor control and motor learning research is publicized through meetings of NASPSPA, in many of the sport psychology journals mentioned previously, in eclectic publications such as *Quest*, the *Journal of Human Movement Studies*, and the *Research Quarterly for Exercise and Sport*, and in journals specifically designed to focus on motor learning, such as the *Journal of Motor Behavior*, *Motor Skills*, *Theory into Practice*, and *Perceptual and Motor Skills*.

## A LOOK TO THE FUTURE

Sport sociology, sport psychology, motor development and motor learning, emerged during the latter part of the 20th century as ways to understand human movement phenomena, particularly sport, through the theories and methods of the social sciences. In the process, they have tended to divide and isolate aspects of human performance into discrete academic territories confined within disciplinary boundaries. Although this specialization may lead to invaluable insights, it tends to fragment understanding and dislocate the discipline. Recent scholarship seems to suggest trends toward interdisciplinary integration, a broader focus, applied analysis and utilitarian understandings, liberal learning skills, curricular collusion and cooption, and examining multiculturalism and movement.

## A Trend Toward Interdisciplinary Integration

A premise of contemporary kinesiology is the integration of diverse disciplinary approaches into the holistic study of humans moving. This renaissance breadth of vision, which is the desired product of the liberal arts approach to the study of movement, counteracts the pinching narrowness of some aspects of the traditional curriculum. Kinesiology is new and is evolving rapidly. Its interdisciplinary potential is still relatively untapped. Within the social sciences, kinesiology dwells not only in the mainstream of each subject field, but also in the intersections between subjects such as sociology and psychology (social psychology) and uses whichever methodologies seem most illuminating for a given project. Rather than running the risk of getting isolated within subject boundaries, kinesiology stresses the connections and holistic meanings.

To fully understand the social significance of modern sport, for example, mainstream psychology, sociology, and anthropology are supplemented with insights from the overlapping intersections of these fields and also from other social science subject areas. Economic theory illuminates the marketplace of sport. Political science theories help kinesiology students appreciate the institutional qualities of sport, its governance system, and its relationship with other cultural institutions. The role and functioning of sport in international politics is informed by current international relations theory. Knowledge of economics, political science, and international relations forms a basis for addressing complex multifaceted issues such as the extent to which sport is either pluralistic or hegemonic in nature, and public policy questions concerning the future directions of sport.

Interdisciplinary integration applies beyond the realm of the social sciences. As recent developments in motor learning and sport psychology suggest, these connections span the arts and the sciences. In his prognosis for future lines of research in cognitive aspects of motor learning and performance, Christina (1987) suggested:

*In the future we should use an interdisciplinary approach and incorporate ideas and methods from biomechanics and a number of other fields, which collectively may be referred to as cognitive science. (p. 31)*

Among these collaborating fields he included philosophy, computer science, linguistics, and neuroscience, as well as anthropology and psychology. Similarly, contemporary sport psychology features collaboration between, and integration of, a range of disciplinary approaches in an endeavor to better understand human movement behavior. Harris (1987) described six major frontiers of exercise and sport psychology, each of which crosses traditional disciplinary boundaries:

1. knowledge of the brain.
2. psychophysiological approaches.
3. psychobiological approaches.
4. self-regulation.
5. educational sport psychology and service.
6. social psychological approaches.

No less important are the initiatives to integrate approaches appropriated from the humanities and social sciences to study human movement.

In the greater arena of higher education, divisions between the humanities and social sciences have become blurred (as indicated by the spate of recent articles in the *Chronicle of Higher Education* (Geertz, 1980; Scully, 1980; Winkler, 1985, 1987a, 1987b; Coughlin, 1987; Paul, 1988). Responsive to trends within the educational enterprise, of which it is a part, contemporary kinesiology is responding by emphasizing the interdisciplinary study of physical activity and performance. MacAloon (1984), a leading advocate of interdisciplinary rapprochement as exemplified in his own scholarship, recognized this trend toward the future:

*Broader communities of scholars will discover in the performance approach an answer to that most important intellectual challenge of the next decades: the opening of new lines of contact between the humanities and social sciences. (p. 5)*

## A Trend Toward a Broader Focus

The frontiers of exercise and sport psychology, summarized by Harris (1987), highlight a second, no less important, feature of contemporary kinesiology: its integrative inclusivity. Traditional physical education programs too often had been narrowed to the study of sport and, in particular, elite performance within sport. Adopting human movement in every form, at all performance levels, and throughout the lifespan as the focus of kinesiology (discussed in chapter 2) has implications for the undergraduate curriculum and the research agenda. The frontiers that Harris envisioned reach to the interrelationship of brain functions from psychological, physiological, and biological perspectives. These have ramifications for human movement behavior beyond the sports field. Research on self-regulation, for instance, certainly will impact the sphere of supportive movement if and when it becomes possible to regulate stress levels and self-treat psychosomatic diseases through autonomic physiological methods such as biofeedback. Likewise, motor learning is expanding its scope and mission to include all forms of movement. Christina (1987) suggested that in contemporary motor learning:

*We need to extend our applied research beyond the boundaries of sport to lines of research in other areas such as gerontology and health and physical rehabilitation. (p. 34)*

## A Trend Toward Applied Analysis and Utilitarian Understandings

Contemporary kinesiologists are aware of two imperatives for the field.

1. Broadening the scope of kinesiology to all forms of movement.
2. Recognizing the utilitarian value of applied knowledge.

Although a liberal arts approach to studying human movement is not premised or dependent upon any one professional outlet for its validation, it nevertheless is concerned with understanding, changing, and even improving "the real world." Even during the pursuit of knowledge for its own sake, kinesiology students recognize the humanitarian services that can be rendered through human movement professions. Through their study and research they could advance knowledge at the frontiers of research identified by Harris and others. Subsequently, as professionals in the field, they could apply this information for the betterment of young and old, healthy and infirm, throughout every strata of the population, to "alter the likelihood that people will live higher quality lives and that the nation's stock of human capital will be improved" (Ellis, 1990, p. 13).

## A Trend Toward Liberating Liberal Learning Skills

An aim of the liberal arts approach to kinesiology is to develop learning skills that are liberating and that will help the student become an independent learner. Each of the social sciences may contribute to the critical sensitivity and cultural awareness of the kinesiology undergraduate, but none as much as sociocultural studies. By analyzing the distribution and allocation of resources, economic and cultural control, social stratification and power, students are better equipped to understand a range of issues that pertain to human movement and health care, the environment and sport. Through critical sociological imagination, kinesiology undergraduates are better prepared to serve their community as a member of one of the human movement professions. Similarly, through experiencing on a firsthand basis the potentialities of their own bodies by participating in a range of physical activities, graduating students are better equipped to cope, care, and cure in their future vocations.

## A Trend Toward Curricular Collusion and Cooption

In the interests of integration and cooperation, contemporary kinesiology stresses collusion and even cooption whenever that curricular option is viable. Rather than continuing the process of splintering knowledge into subfields, contemporary kinesiology urges combining expertise. Through collaboration across traditional subject barriers, kinesiologists explore the interstices between hitherto discrete subject areas. Indications are that steps toward streamlining the social sciences in kinesiology are being considered. The precedent set in Europe of combining the psychology of activity and motor learning into one field has encouraged many innovators to develop a collusive international curriculum that conforms to the European example. A second initiative designed to integrate kinesiology is that of cooption: the implementation of a developmental approach throughout the field and the dismantling of the subdiscipline of motor development. As Thomas and Thomas (1989) have suggested:

*All courses in human movement should be taught from a developmental perspective, research should be done within the appropriate subdiscipline, and some of that research should be developmental. Motor development will be best served if researchers align with scientists within the subdisciplines and share developmental information in cross-disciplinary groups. (p. 203)*

## A Trend Toward Examining Multiculturalism and Movement

The anthropological avenue of analysis seldom has been developed systematically and rigorously within kinesiology. Yet, as information technology, telecommunications, and access to transportation shrink the world by bringing diverse cultures together, kinesiology is empowered to serve the global community through the study of cultural diversity in human movement. Physical activity is a universal phenomenon; sport spans the globe. At its peak, in athletic festivals such as the Olympic Games, it becomes a universal language, a dialogue between individual participants and between national identities. Even as technological possibilities tend to bring world communities together, recognition of cultural differences often creates international stereotyping and divisive prejudice as people judge others from the perspective of their own cultural upbringing. The cross-cultural study of human movement helps to overcome this ethnocentrism.

Through participation in, and appreciation of, mutually agreeable, inherently nonthreatening physical pastimes, cultural differences are studied, international similarities noted, and multiculturalism facilitated. The purpose of cross-cultural study is not to construct some homogenized universal identity but, rather, to develop recognition, respect, and accommodation of individual and cultural difference. Multicultural sensitivity goes beyond tolerance of foreign habits in foreign places to recognition and respect for the expression of a multiplicity of ethnic identities within one's own society. This recognition invokes two forms of respect:

*Respect for the unique identities of each individual regardless of gender, race, or ethnicity and respect for those activities, practices, and ways of viewing the world that are particularly valued by, or associated with, members of disadvantaged groups. (Gutmann, et al., 1992, p. 8)*

Although neither cultural anthropology nor physical anthropology has achieved mainstream status in kinesiology, there are signs that the universal significance of human movement and multicultural awareness are impinging on the consciousness of the profession. Park (1991) summarized this trend:

*The addition in 1982 of cultural anthropology to the sociology section of the* Research Quarterly for Exercise and Sport, *and the increasing use of participant observation and ethnographic techniques in studying physical education classes, sports settings, and health and exercise preferences of different populations, will enable this much neglected aspect of our work to grow. (p. 249)*

## APPRECIATING HUMAN MOVEMENT THROUGH THE HUMANITIES

The humanities, which together with the social sciences and the natural sciences comprise a liberal education, provide unique contributions to the study of humans moving. They reach beyond clinical examination of the principles underlying human movement to provide depth, color, and texture to the appreciation of physical activity. The humanities enable a holistic understanding of the humanistic dimensions of movement phenomena.

The main disciplines in the humanities are philosophy, religion, history (which also may be constituted as a social science), literature, the fine arts, and the performing arts. Under these general categories fall several well established academic approaches, many of which have been appropriated by kinesiology to illuminate humans moving (as illustrated in Figure 6.2).

The discussion in chapter 4 stressed the importance of *philosophy* in kinesiology — in particular, developing a philosophical framework within which to operate, learning to think critically and reflectively about fundamental questions of knowledge and value, and learning to develop and exercise the powers of logical analysis, creative imagination, and evaluative judgment. The subarea of philosophy that is particularly enlightening in the context of expressive and performative human movement is aesthetics, "the theory or philosophy of taste" (Zeigler, 1990, p. 62).

*Religion* properly belongs with other humanities because they, in contrast to the sciences, are all concerned principally with the critical study of human ideas and values. The relationships among play, sport, and religion are awakening considerable interest in contemporary

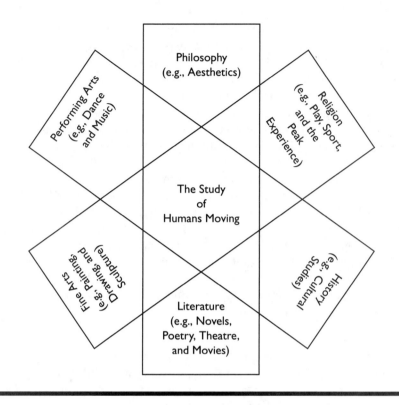

**FIGURE 6.2**

Humanities and Humans Moving

scholars. Hoffman (1992), editor of *Sport and Religion*, noted some of the similarities:

*Each, for example, stirs passions deep in the human spirit, and each can have profound and enduring effects on the individual and on society. Both offer unique windows into the collective social conscience. Understanding the forms of play and the religious life of a society furthers one's understanding of the values, motivations, and character of its people. (p. vii)*

*History* provides context, an understanding of the evolution of kinesiology (the subject of section 3), and an awareness of cultural history. From the distant realms of Ancient Greece and Rome, encountered through courses in classical civilizations, to more recent developments in modern culture, examined in programs such as American Studies, history illuminates a broad range of human movement phenomena.

*Literature* provides insights into the lived experience of physical activity through various genres. These range from poetry to novels, from fictional accounts to nonfictional biographies, from theatre to cinema. Examining the western physical experience through literature can be augmented in comparative literature courses including books, plays, poems, and films conceived in other cultures, which provide insight into the experience of human movement.

The *fine arts* often have gravitated toward the human body and its movement patterns as a subject of their creative expression. In paintings, drawings, prints, and sculpture through the ages, the active human body and, in particular, the elite athlete has been well represented in and through art. The performing art of especial relevance to kinesiology is *dance*. Through various forms of dance popular in an array of cultures, kinesiology students study expressive and performative movement from around the world. Dance forms range from the formal approaches of ballet to the creative expression of modern dance, from social to folk dance, and from archaic, once popular, dance forms to ultracontemporary forms of dance. In every case, the other prominent performing art, *music*, plays an integral part in the process of creative expression through dance.

## A LOOK BACK

The humanities have been represented sparingly in most physical education programs of the past. Although history and philosophy usually have found a place in the curriculum, they rarely have been tapped to clarify the nature of the creative, expressive, or performative movement processes. Where the humanities found a niche in the curriculum, they did so under the aegis of sports studies. History, philosophy, and literature have illuminated the nature of sport and the significance of the sport experience. Each of these three subfields has evolved to such a level of organizational formality that each now has an organization and at least one journal.

The first meeting of the National Society for Sport History (NSSH) took place in 1973. This organization publishes the *Journal of Sport History*. The other major periodical for scholars working in that field is the *Canadian Journal of History of Sport and Physical Education*.

In the same year as the inauguration of NSSH, the Philosophic Society for the Study of Sport (PSSS) was formed. Its founding fathers were a group of philosophers with an interest in sport who were in attendance at the annual meeting of the American Philosophical Association as well as some physical educators interested in philosophy. This society published its first issue of the *Journal of the Philosophic Society for the Study of Sport* in 1974. Sport history and sport philosophy both are represented in the formal structure of the national governing body of the allied fields of human movement in the United States: The American Alliance of Health, Physical Education, Recreation and Dance

(AAHPERD). The sport history academy and the sport philosophy academy of the National Association of Sport and Physical Education (NASPE) meet annually at the national AAHPERD conventions.

The field of sport literature is of more recent origin. Faculty in English and in physical education joined to form the Sport Literature Association (SLA) in 1982. In 1983, the association published the first issue of *Arete: The Journal of Sport Literature*. *Arete* subsequently was retitled *Aethlon* to avoid confusing it with another journal of the same name.

Recent scholarship seems to suggest certain trends in the humanities: toward expansion and integration, appreciation of the lived experience, aesthetic education, physical literature, and physical literacy.

## A LOOK TO THE FUTURE

## A Trend Toward Expansion and Integration

Sport is such a ubiquitous phenomenon in western culture that it merits a niche within kinesiology. In addition, scholarship within the humanities, which has tended to confine itself rather narrowly to elite athletic performance is expanding to encompass sport at all levels of performance, more functional supportive physical activity, and expressive and performative movement. In the past, a student considering entry into kinesiology, motivated perhaps by an interest in fitness and a concern for health, would have felt disenfranchised by a singular scholarly preoccupation with sport. Expanding humanistic elements of the curriculum to incorporate the spectrum of human movement experience is empowering for such a student.

Interdisciplinary integration facilitates the juxtaposition of thematic constructs, one against the other, in ways that are likely to produce insights into the human movement experience. For example, consideration of religion and physical activity inevitably will lead to contemplation of the peak experience (Maslow, 1968; Ravizza, 1984; Ryan, 1986), or of the religious qualities of play (Moltmann, 1972; Sheehan, 1978), or of the relationship between sport and religion (Guttman, 1978; Novak, 1976). To deepen awareness of religion, sport, and self, interdisciplinary integration extends beyond the confines of the humanities to incorporate perspectives from both the natural sciences and the social sciences. In addition to ideas from religion, literature, philosophy, history, cultural studies, and popular culture, kinesiology can take ideas from social sciences such as sociology, psychology, and anthropology. As Hoffman (1992) predicted:

*Those willing to examine sport and religion through multidisciplinary lenses and to supplement their vision through recollections of personal experiences in their sporting and religious lives will be rewarded with a fresh and stimulating view of a fascinating aspect of American society. (p. viii)*

Similar cross-referencing from one field of study to another may illuminate the human element of physical experiences.

## A Trend Toward Appreciation of the Lived Experience

Since the 1960s, the study of human movement has become more research oriented, scholarly, and fragmented. As a result, "whole-person scholarship" has tended to fall through the cracks between subdisciplines until recently. With increasing awareness that specialization has dissected the human experience into discipline-manageable segments (Ellis, 1988; Newell, 1990; Lawson, 1991), the humanistic dimensions of physical activity are receiving renewed interest (Harris, 1989; Hellison, 1991). Each of the humanities disciplines presents unique opportunities for appreciating the physical sensations, the emotional feelings, and the context of physical activity experiences. Art, for example, teaches the visual appreciation of movement; literature offers insights into areas of life beyond the ring, the court, and the field; and philosophy provides aesthetic appreciation.

## A Trend Toward Aesthetic Education

In clinically examining and analyzing human movement, the intrinsic joy and beauty of the experience are easily overlooked. Aesthetic education redresses this imbalance by fostering "disinterested and sympathetic attention to and contemplation of any object of awareness whatever, for its own sake alone" (Stolnitz, 1960, p. 35). Through all modes of perception — sight, taste, touch, sound, smell, and the kinesthetic sense — the abilities to appreciate and discriminate are refined. The affinity between aesthetic appreciation and physical activity is seen in the intrinsic artistic nature of the experience. Peter Arnold (1988), a British philosopher, has suggested that:

*It is possible to divide physical activities up into three logically separate categories: (i) those sports that are non-aesthetic; (ii) those sports that are partially aesthetic; (iii) those activities such as dance and mime that can be considered art. (p. 77)*

In each of these categories beauty abounds, but as the aesthetic purpose and artistic performance become more highly accentuated, the skills of aesthetic appreciation assume proportional significance. In the cases of sports, such as football, boxing, and ice hockey, as examples, beauty is of incidental significance, whereas in sports such as gymnastics, diving, skating, synchronized swimming, and surfing, the form of the performance becomes a paramount consideration. At the higher end of the aesthetic spectrum are movement forms such as dance and mime, which are premised upon the foundations of art. They deliberately set out to evoke an aesthetic response in spectators. As artistic compositions they combine creative form with the performer's disciplined expression to evoke images and responses through a visual spectacle.

Physical activity in general, and sport in particular, are vested with significant meanings for many students. Literature, defined broadly to include popular culture such as movies, has depicted the trials, tribulations, joys, and successes of people struggling to succeed in sport and to overcome physical debilitation. Early examples from the various genres are drama (such as Arthur Miller's *Death of a Salesman*), novels (such as *Rabbit Run* by John Updike), non-fiction prose (such as John McPhee's *Levels of the Game*) and poetry (such as *Morning Athletes* by Marge Piercy).

Perhaps the greatest groundswell of popular literature is taking place in the predilection of movie-makers for themes featuring the physical experience (often taken from best-selling novels such as Bernard Malamud's *The Natural*). Ever since the *Chariots of Fire* won national acclaim (and box-office success), movies are increasingly raising important questions about life in sensitive ways. These movies include *Hoosiers*, *Field of Dreams*, and *A League of Their Own*. Movies such as *A River Runs Through It* discuss significant themes such as religion and environmental awareness through a lens of recreational pastimes (the tone adopted in the movie is taken from Normal MacLean's best selling poetic reminiscence, which begins, "In our family there was no clear line between religion and fly fishing"). Others, such as *My Left Foot*, portray the human struggle against physical limitation. As contemporary literature begins to mine the rich veins of sportive and supportive movement for serious material, kinesiology would be remiss if it were to fail to respond.

The plethora of excellent literature of all forms, highlighting the human physical experiences, is a resource for kinesiology students. Through guided exposure to this literature, students learn to appreciate the form, style, and technique of transmitting meanings through language and images. Well selected literature reflects or scrutinizes national beliefs and values, captures a wide range of social and psychological conditions, and examines moral and ethical behavior. By including literature in the curriculum, kinesiology programs contribute to one of the central goals of higher education, that of expanding cultural literacy.

Words represent only a small proportion of the total range of human communication. The human body has immense expressive potential. Yet higher education emphasizes the verbal mode of expression. Through informed observation, students can better understand the symbolic components of an individual's movement. Given the extraordinary complexity of body language (defined by Moore & Yamamoto, 1993), in *Beyond Words* as "a multifaceted, constantly changing nonlinear form of communication" p. 285), interpreting movement messages is fraught with difficulties. Not the least of the many problems in deciphering the meanings is that "a given action may convey, at one and the same time, multiple meanings, some that are pan-human, others that are culture-specific, and still others that are singularly individualistic" (p. 285). Building upon the movement analysis of Rudolph Laban (1974), Moore and Yamamoto are among many scholars from fields such as kinesiology, anthropology, psychology, and neuropsychology working to unravel the mysteries of physical expression. The field is in its infancy, as Moore and Yamamoto conclude:

*Body movement is the first seat of knowledge for the human child. So too it was the first source of knowledge for the species. It would therefore seem we should know a great deal about human movement. But what we do not yet know is greater still. Perhaps as we continue to explore the world beyond words, we may lift the veil of ignorance a little more and, by so doing, illuminate not only where we have been but also where we are going. (p. 297)*

## EXPERIENCING HUMAN MOVEMENT

*Kinesiology without participation in movement activities is like a music program in which no one ever plays an instrument. (Bain, 1991, p. 216)*

Linda Bain's (1991) metaphor captures the feeling of the many kinesiology departments nationwide that incorporate physical activities into their programs. In kinesiology, the study of movement is supplemented by study *through* movement. Physical activity classes should occupy an important niche in any curriculum, but too often they have been a trapping, even an embarrassment, to the academic faculty. As Bain (1991) noted, "It is ironic that a field that focuses on human movement has deemphasized the 'body knowledge' that comes from directly experiencing movement" (p. 216). Classes offered as a service to the student body often have been perceived and treated as less important than the concentration in kinesiology. This relegation of activity classes to secondary status often has been accompanied by a willingness to delegate responsibility for their teaching to campus recreation, adjunct, part-time faculty, and even graduate students. In recent years, however, the scholastic distinction between the life of the mind and the education of the body have been challenged. Some even have suggested that movement, sport, and exercise cannot be studied usefully except within environmental contexts (Martens, 1967). In the wake of this changing attitude, many kinesiology departments nationwide are instituting physical activity programs that meet the cognitive, affective, and psychomotor goals of a liberal education.

The dual premise of a liberal arts physical activity curriculum is *symbiosis* and *integration*, the notion that the mind and the body, the intellectual and the physical are mutually dependent. Too frequently, education tends to compartmentalize the life of the mind away from the experience of the body. Contemporary theorists are increasingly espousing holistic approaches, ones that promote the unity of being over any conceptually schizophrenic curriculum model. As an alternative to the disintegration of the learning experience caused by departmental boundaries, physical activities foster the integration of disciplines through a unified focus on learning in and through environmental contexts. For example, in the case of outdoor education, nature is an ideal laboratory. Students learn instinctively in this laboratory, and, in addition, these lessons of nature can be integrated with the wisdom of the classroom to foster deep and uniquely integrative learning experiences.

Many experiential education advocates embrace the philosophy of John Dewey as they devise situations in which their students learn by doing. This approach can be refined and extended to structure the learning experience at the most intellectual level. Established academic disciplines and emerging fields of study provide a wealth of resources and ideas that are being applied to the outdoor adventure experience to both enlighten and enrich the participants. The outdoor adventure has multidisciplinary ramifications, revealed through the trinity of the liberal arts: the humanities, the social sciences, and the natural sciences.

Just as a laboratory experience provides a unique tactile and problem-solving dimension to a science class, an activity class can be structured to illustrate academic subject matter. For example, a weight-training class can be designed to study the musculoskeletal system taught in human anatomy classes. Students come to appreciate the origin, location and insertion of each muscle, and to see and experience muscles in action. Other examples of integrating science and the outdoor experience are studies of the biomechanics of the body's lever systems when rock climbing and the physiology of hypothermia when backpacking. The psychology of risk taking, the sociology of group dynamics, and the anthropology of the play patterns and relationships of primitive tribes with their environment — all take on added meaning when they are taught in and through a lifetime activity or a sporting experience.

Just like the social sciences, the humanities assume new, more directly challenging proportions when removed from the distant realms of textbooks and classrooms to the immediately relevant context of personal experience. The naturalistic literature and transcendental philosophy of Wordsworth, Thoreau, and Emerson resonate better in natural surroundings than within the four walls of a lecture hall. The artistic landscapes of Constable and the athletic sculptures of R. Tait McKenzie come to life when juxtaposed against their sources of inspiration. Consideration of the relationship with nature of eastern religions such as Shinto and Zen Buddhism assumes a different level of meaning in a natural environment. The intellectual dimensions of physical activity are limited only by the imagination and expertise involved in designing these classes.

Often, the *intellectual* meanings depend upon personal experiences. For instance, aesthetics can be observed from a distance without its being really understood. Only when learning through experience can students become truly aesthetically educated.

*The aesthetically educated person is not so much the person who is able to talk about, describe, or comment upon certain objects and situations in a certain way as the person who in fact has a capacity for experiencing, understanding and becoming involved with them. (Collinson, 1973, p. 197)*

Applying the theory of *aesthetics* to a range of practical experience from competitive sport to dance brings meaning and relevance to conceptual cognition. It becomes more than an exercise in ideas, more like preparation for a fulfilling life.

*Aesthetic education consists centrally in the cultivating of an individual's capacity to regard things, including things which he himself might have made or be making or performing, with a particular kind of imaginative attention and to become increasingly discriminating and critically reflective in his responses to them. (Redfern, 1986, p. 67)*

The *affective* impact of experiential learning far exceeds the intellectual study of a movement form without participation in it. Concerning the medium of dance, Arnold (1988) observed:

*In the harmonious blending of motion with emotion, the dancer is able to realize himself as few others have the power to do. What is felt and meaningfully constituted, although sometimes capable of being described in words, is not reducible to words. Its 'meaningfulness' lies in its own mode of expression. (p. 143)*

Physical activities are included in the curriculum to foster intellectual understanding, aesthetic appreciation, and affective involvement. An array of lifetime skills, adventure activities, and sporting opportunities brings with it a spectrum of learning and emotional experiences: from joy, fulfillment, and excitement to fear, frustration, and a sense of limitation. Physical activities also are included in the kinesiology curriculum to develop psychomotor skills. Programs of physical activity traditionally have been justified on the basis of reaching a certain level of competence in the acquisition of skills. This rationale has been particularly persuasive in programs designed to prepare students to teach. The ability to model a skill, demonstrate effectively and incisively analyze and synthesize the movement patterns of school children is inextricably linked with the teacher's skill level and understanding. Kinesiology students selecting careers other than teaching also should be exposed to a range of movement forms. Competence in lifetime and outdoor activities, team and individual sports, aquatic activities, and dance are essential components of a contemporary kinesiology program. As Jerry Thomas (1990), a past president of the American Academy of Kinesiology and Physical Education, summarized the rationale for requiring all kinesiology students to experience sportive activity: "One who has no expertise in a sport cannot study the skilled nature of the behavior satisfactorily" (p. 11).

Regardless of the level of performance students may reach during the program of activity, kinesiologists will learn to empathize with future clients through the struggle to move effectively, efficiently, and even superbly. For example, an aspiring physical therapist in an undergraduate kinesiology program will be better prepared through personal experience with physical adversity, through the challenges of adventure education, and through the experience of success in physical activity classes than through the solitary medium of book learning.

Understanding psychomotor efficiency through wellness-related courses in exercise physiology, nutrition, and the psychology of exercise is an important foundation for any student aspiring to be employed within the human movement and allied health professions. In a complete kinesiology program, conceptual recognition is accompanied by curricular implementation. Through activity courses students are given the opportunity to reach a desired level of health-related physical fitness and to surpass a minimum level of cardiovascular and muscular fitness and flexibility. Thomas (1990) represents the view of many in the kinesiology profession in his assertion, "It is a reasonable expectation that people who study movement should have and maintain an acceptable level of health-related physical fitness" (p. 11).

## SUMMARY

During undergraduate preparation, students of kinesiology should be exposed to three pillars of wisdom. The foundation of one's future is a personal *philosophy*. Throughout a career and personal life, every decision individuals make is premised upon a philosophical conviction. These principles should be developed carefully in and through the kinesiology concentration. In the second pillar, the *science of human movement*, every student of kinesiology should emerge from an undergraduate program with a clear idea of how and why people move. This scientific foundation provides the basis for continued study and professional applications that help people move more effectively (e.g., teaching, coaching, sport research) or to overcome hindrances to movement efficiency (e.g., various forms of therapy and medicine). The third pillar in this foundational tripod, the *humanistic dimension* of physical activity, addresses the study of the human mover. Every movement has personal meaning. A holistic approach to kinesiology is premised upon an understanding of humans moving. This knowledge may be acquired in part from the study of the social sciences and the humanities. The explanatory power of personal experience offers additional insights: "One important aspect of alternative ways of knowing is legitimating experiential knowledge" (Bain, 1991, p. 216). A comprehensive, challenging, and diverse physical activity program fosters appreciation of what it means to be a human being moving.

The conceptual emphasis upon the qualitative aspects of the physical experience represents a shift in emphasis that many leading scholars in the field see as being essential to the future health of kinesiology. Susan Greendorfer (1991) addressed this question in a paper presented at the 1990 Annual Meeting of the American Academy of Kinesiology and Physical Education:

*Equally as critical, . . . is the necessity to shift our paradigmatic focus to a more broadly based conceptual structure — one more inclusive then the biologistic conceptualization that historically underlies our thinking. An expanded knowledge structure that incorporates identity, intention, influence, ideology, interaction, context, and expression offers the promise of a new direction. Without these integral concepts embedded firmly in our conceptualization of subject matter, we will not have integration; nor will we begin to develop terms, definitions, and concepts that are mutually understood and agreed upon. (p. 53, 54)*

# REFERENCES

Arnold, P. J. (1979). *Meaning in movement, sport and physical education.* London: Heinemann.

Arnold, P. J. (1988). *Education, movement and the curriculum.* New York: Falmer Press.

Bain, L. L. (1991). Further reactions to Newell: Knowledge as contested terrain. *Quest, 43*(2), 214-217.

Christina, R. W. (1987). Motor learning: Future lines of research. In *American Academy of Physical Education Papers* (Vol. 20, pp. 214-217). Champaign, IL: Human Kinetics.

Colfer, G. R., Hamilton, K. E., Magill, R. A., & Hamilton, B. J. (1986). *Contemporary physical education.* Dubuque, IA: Wm. C. Brown.

Collinson, D. (1973). Aesthetic education. In G. Langford & D. J. O'Conner (Eds), *New essays in the philosophy of education.* London: Routledge and Kegan Paul.

Coughlin, E. K. (September 2, 1987). Humanities and social sciences: The sound of barriers falling. *Chronicle of Higher Education,* pp. A6, A7, A10, A12.

Ellis, M. J. (1988). Warning: The pendulum has swung far enough. *Journal of Physical Education, Recreation and Dance, 59,* 75-78.

Ellis, M. J. (1990). Reactions to "The Body of Knowledge: A Common Core." In *American Academy of Physical Education Papers* (pp. 13-16). Champaign, IL: Human Kinetics.

Geertz, C. (1980). Blurred genes: The refiguration of social thought. *American Scholar, 49,* 165-179.

Greendorfer, S. L. (1991). New directions or the same old problem. In *American Academy of Physical Education Papers,* (Vol 24, pp. 48-55). Champaign, IL: Human Kinetics.

Guttmann, A. (1978). *From ritual to record: The nature of modern sports.* New York: Columbia University Press.

Gutmann, A., Taylor, D., Rockefeller, S., Walzer, M., & Wolf, S. (1992). *Multiculturalism and "The politics of recognition."* Princeton, NJ: Princeton University Press.

Harris, D. V. (1987). Frontiers in psychology of exercise and sport. In *American Academy of Physical Education Papers,* (Vol. 20, pp. 42-52). Champaign, IL: Human Kinetics.

Harris, J. C. (1989). Suited up and stripped down: Perspectives for sociocultural sports studies. *Sociology of Sport Journal, 6,* 335-347.

Hellison, D. (1991). The whole person in physical education scholarship: Toward integration. *Quest, 43* (1991), 307-318.

Hoffman, S. J. (Ed.). (1992). *Sport and religion.* Champaign, IL: Human Kinetics.

Kenyon, G. S., & Loy, J. W. (1965). Toward a sociology of sport. *Journal of Health, Physical Education and Recreation, 36,* 5, 24-25, 68-69.

Laban, R. (1974). *The language of movement.* Boston: Plays, Inc.

Latash, M. L. (1993). *Control of human movement.* Champaign, IL: Human Kinetics.

Lawson, H. A. (1991). Specialization and fragmentation among faculty as endemic features of academic life. *Quest, 43* (1991), 280-295.

MacAloon, J. J. (1984). Introduction: Cultural performances, culture theory. In J. J. MacAloon (Ed.), *Rite, drama, festival, spectacle: Rehearsals toward a theory of cultural performance* (pp. 1-15). Philadelphia: Institute for the Study of Human Issues.

Martens, R. (1987). Science, knowledge, and sport psychology. *Sport Psychologist, 1,* 29-55.

Maslow, A. (1968). *Toward a psychology of being* (2nd ed.). New York: Van Nostrand Reinhold.

McPherson, B. D., Curtis, J. E., & Loy, J. W. (1989). *The social significance of sport: An introduction to the sociology of sport.* Champaign, IL: Human Kinetics.

Moltmann, J. (1972). *Theology of play.* New York: Harper.

Moore, C. L., & Yamamoto, K. (1993). *Beyond words: Movement observation and analysis.* Philadelphia: Gordon & Brach.

Newell, K. M. (1990). Physical education in higher education: Chaos out of order. *Quest, 42,* 227-242.

Novak, M. (1976). *The joy of sports: End zones, bases, baskets, balls, and the consecration of the American spirit.* New York: Basic Books.

Park, R. J. (1991). On tilting at windmills while facing Armageddon. *Quest, 43,* 247-259.

Paul, A. (1988, February 10). Writing about writing: Leading anthropologist casts a literary eye on classic works in his field. *Chronicle of Higher Education,* pp. A4, A6.

Ravizza, K. (1984). Qualities of the peak experience in sport. In J. M. Silva & R. S. Weinberg (Eds), *Psychological foundations of sport* (pp. 535-544). Champaign, IL: Human Kinetics.

Redfern, H. B. (1986). *Questions in aesthetic education.* London: Allen and Unwin.

Ryan, T. (1986). *Wellness, spirituality and sports.* Mahweh, NJ: Paulist Press.

Sage, G. S. (1990). *Power and ideology in American sport.* Champaign, IL: Human Kinetics.

Scully, M. G. (1980, March 31). Social scientists, unable to explain some issues, turning to humanists. *Chronicle of Higher Education,* pp. 1-5.

Sheehan, G. (1978). *Running and being.* New York: Warner Books.

Stolnitz, J. (1960). *Aesthetics and philosophy of art criticism.* New York: Houghton Mifflin.

Thomas, J. R. (1990). The body of knowledge: A common core. In *American Academy of Physical Education Papers* (Vol. 23, pp. 5-12). Champaign, IL: Human Kinetics.

Thomas, J. R., & Thomas, K. T. (1989). What is motor development? Where does it belong? *Quest, 41,* 203.

Updike, J. (1960). *Rabbit Run.* New York: Fawcett.

Winkler, K. J. (1985, June 26). Questioning the science in social science: Scholars signal a "turn to interpretation." *Chronicle of Higher Education,* pp. 5-6.

Winkler, K. J. (1987a, October 7). Interdisciplinary research: How big a challenge to traditional fields? *Chronicle of Higher Education* pp. A1, A15.

Winkler, K. J. (1987b, November 25). Post-structuralism: An often-abstruse French import profoundly affects research in the United States. *Chronicle of Higher Education,* pp. A6-A8.

Zeigler, E. F. (1990). *Sport and physical education: Past, present, future.* Champaign, IL: Stipes Publishing.

## SUGGESTED READING

Albrecht, L., & Brewer, R. (Eds.) (1990). *Bridges of Power: Women's Multicultural Alliances.* Santa Cruz, CA: New Society Publishers.

Allison, L. (1986). *The Politics of Sport.* Manchester, IN: Manchester University Press.

Bale, J. (1989). *Sports Geography.* New York: E. and F. N. Spon.

Bandura, A. (1986) *Social Foundations of Thought and Action: A Social Cognitive Theory.* Englewood Cliffs, NJ: Prentice Hall.

Clark, J., & Humphrey, J. (1985). *Motor Development.* Princeton, NJ: Princeton University Press.

Coakley, J. J. (1990). *Sport in Society: Issues and Controversies.* St. Louis: Times Mirror/Mosby.

Corbin, C. (Ed.). (1980). *A Textbook of Motor Development.* Dubuque, IA: Wm. C. Brown.

Dunleavy, A. O., Miracle, A. W., & Rees, C. R. (Eds.). (1982). *Studies in The Sociology of Sport.* Fort Worth, TX: Texas Christian University Press.

Elias, N., & Dunning, E. (1986). *Quest For Excitement.* Oxford: Blackwell.

Espenchade, A. S., & Eckerts, H. M. (1980). *Motor Development.* Columbus, OH: Charles E. Merrill.

Figler, S. K., & Whitaker, G. (1991). *Sport and Play in American Life.* Dubuque, IA: Wm. C. Brown.

Giammalti, A. B. (1989). *Take Time For Paradise: Americans and Their Games.* New York: Summit Books.

Gill, D. L. (1986). *Psychological Dynamics of Sport.* Champaign, IL: Human Kinetics.

Green, M., & Jenkins, C. (Eds.). (1982). *Sporting Fictions.* Birmingham, U.K.: University of Birmingham, Centre for Contemporary Cultural Studies.

Greendorfer, S. L., & Yiannakis, A. (Eds.). (1981). *Sociology of Sport: Diverse Perspectives.* West Point, NY: Leisure Press.

Gruneau, R. (1983). *Class, Sports and Social Development.* Amherst, MA: University of Massachusetts Press.

Hargreaves, J. (1986). *Sport, Power and Culture.* New York: St. Masters Press.

Hargreaves, J. (Ed.). (1982). *Sports, Culture and Ideology.* London: Routledge and Kegan Paul.

Harris, J. C., & Park, R. J. (Eds.). (1983). *Play, Games and Sports in Cultural Contexts.* Champaign, IL: Human Kinetics.

Harvey, J., & Cantelon, M. (Eds.). (1988). *Not Just a Game.* Ottawa: University of Ottawa Press.

Horn, T. S. (Ed.). (1992). *Advances in Sport Psychology.* Champaign, IL: Human Kinetics.

Huizinga, J. (1970). Homo Ludens: *A Study of The Play Element in Culture.* London: Paladin.

Ibrahim, H. (1991). *Leisure and Society: A Comparative Approach.* Dubuque, IA: Wm. C. Brown Publishers.

Ingham, A.. & Loy, J. (Eds.). (1993). *Sport in Social Development: Traditions, Transitions, and Transformations.* Champaign, IL: Human Kinetics.

Kelso, J. A. S., & Clark, J. E. (Eds.). (1982). *The Development of Movement Control and Coordination.* New York: Wiley.

Keogh, J., & Sugden, D. (1985). *Movement Skill Development.* New York: Macmillan.

Kozar, A. J. (1992). *The Sport Sculpture of R. Tait McKenzie.* Champaign, IL: Human Kinetics.

Leonard, W. (1988). *A Sociological Perspective of Sport (3rd ed.).* New York: Macmillan.

Magill, R. A. (Ed.). (1983). *Memory and Control of Action.* Amsterdam: North-Holland.

Magill, R. A. (1993). *Motor Learning: Concepts and Application (4th ed.).* Dubuque, IA: Wm. C. Brown.

Masters, R. (1987). *Coaches Guide to Sport Psychology.* Champaign, IL: Human Kinetics.

Messner, M., & Sabo, D. (Eds.). (1990). *Sport, Men and The Gender Order: Critical Feminist Perspectives.* Champaign, IL: Human Kinetics.

Messner, M. (1992). *Power of Play: Sports and The Problems of Masculinity.* Boston: Beacon Press.

Michener, J. A. (1976). *Sports in America.* New York: Fawcett.

Miles, J. C., & Priest, S. (1990). *Adventure Education.* State College, PA: Venture Publishing Co.

Mitchell, R. (1983). *Mountain Experience: The Psychology and Sociology of Adventure.* Chicago: University of Chicago Press.

Morgan, W. P., & Goldston, S. E. (Eds.). (1987). *Exercise and Mental Health.* New York: Hemisphere.

Mortlock, C. (1984). *The Adventure Alternative*. Cumbria, England: Cicerone.

Nadean, C. H., Halliwell, W. R., Newell, K. M., & Roberts, G. C. (Eds.). (1980). *Psychology of Motor Behavior and Sport*. Champaign, IL: Human Kinetics.

Newell, K. M., & Corcos, D. (Eds.). (1993). *Variability and Motor Control*. Champaign, IL: Human Kinetics.

Nideffer, R. M. (1981). *The Ethics and Practice of Applied Sports Psychology*. Ithaca, NY: Mouvement.

Oriard, M. (1991). *Sporting With The Gods: The Rhetoric of Play and Game in American Culture*. Cambridge, U.K.: Cambridge University Press.

Rarick, G. L. (Ed.) (1973). *Physical Activity: Human Growth and Development*. New York: Academic Press.

Ridenour, M. V. (Ed.). (1978). *Motor Development: Issues and Applications*. Princeton, NJ: Princeton Book Co.

Roberts, G. C. (Ed.). (1992). *Motivation in Sport and Exercise*. Champaign, IL: Human Kinetics.

Schmidt, R. A. (1988). *Motor Control and Learning: A Behavioral Emphasis* (2nd ed.). Champaign, IL: Human Kinetics.

Schmidt, R. A. (1988). *Motor Learning and Performance: From Principles to Practice*. Champaign, IL: Human Kinetics.

Silva, J. M., & Weinberg, R. S. (Eds.). (1984) *Psychological Foundations of Sport*. Champaign, IL: Human Kinetics.

Singer, R. N. (1980). *Motor Learning and Human Performance*. New York: Macmillan.

Straub, W. F. (1978). *Sport Psychology: An Analysis of Athlete Behavior*. Ithaca, NY: Movement.

Telander, R. (1989). *The Hundred Yard Lie*. New York: Fireside.

Theberge, N., & Donnelly, P. (Eds.). (1984). *Sport and The Sociological Imagination*. Fort Worth, TX: Texas Christian University Press.

Toulmin, S. (1972). *Human Understanding*. Princeton, NJ: Princeton University.

Umphlett, W. L. (1975). *The Sporting Myth and The American Experience*. Cranbury, NJ: Associated University Presses.

Vanderwerken, D. L., & Wertz, S. K. (Eds.). (1985). *Sport Inside Out: Readings in Literature and Philosophy*. Fort Worth, TX: Texas Christian University Press.

Weiss, M. R., & Gould, D. (Eds.). (1986). *Sports For Children and Youth*. Champaign, IL: Human Kinetics.

Yiannakis, A., & Greendorfer, S. L. (Eds.). (1992). *Applied Sociology of Sport*. Champaign, IL: Human Kinetics.

*The promise of kinesiology lies in its future, but*
*"A vision of the future depends upon an understanding*
*and intelligent interpretation of the past."*

*(Van Dalen and Bennett, 1971)*

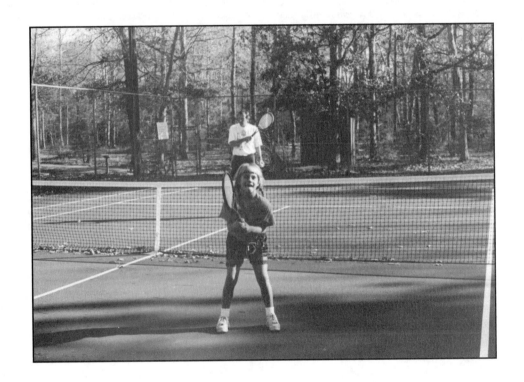

# The Promise of Contemporary Kinesiology

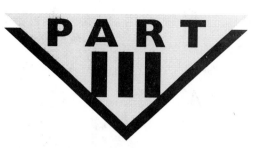

The promise of the kinesiology field of study and profession lies in its future. Paradoxically, though, any evaluation of the future should begin with a look back. As Nevins (1962) suggested:

> Although when we use the word history, we instinctively think of the past, this is an error, for history is actually a bridge connecting the past with the present and pointing the road to the future. (p. 14)

An accurate understanding of the study of human movement in higher education today and all plausible predictions of the future directions of kinesiology are predicated upon informed interpretations of the ideas, events, and individual actions of the past. As Van Dalen and Bennett (1971) concurred in the preface to their *World History of Physical Education*, "A vision of the future depends upon an understanding and intelligent interpretation of the past" (p. viii).

The topic of Chapter 7 is the history of human movement, how this information may be acquired, and where students can find help in the quest for deeper historical insights. Chapter 8, the final chapter, builds upon the historical trends identified in Chapter 7 to assess the future course of kinesiology in higher education and the ways in which a kinesiology graduate can apply the skills and knowledges acquired through a program of study in kinesiology in future professional endeavors.

Nevins, A. (1962). *The gateway to history*. Garden City, NY: Anchor Books.

Van Dalen, D. B., & Bennett, B. (1971). *A world history of physical education*. Englewood Cliffs, NJ: Prentice Hall.

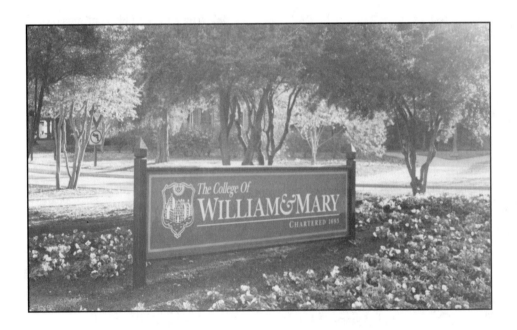

*"A concept of the social forces, conditions, movements, and the philosophers that have come out of the past to shape the institutions of the present day" (Van Dalen & Bennett, 1971)*

# CHAPTER 7

# The History of the Study of Human Movement

The study of human movement is an ongoing process. Events that occur now become history immediately hereafter. Basic ideas, institutions, and cultural movements have shaped this study in the immediate and more distant past. By investigating these seminal events, kinesiology students gain a historical frame of reference, from which to appreciate early happenings in their own context, understand the impact of these events on the current state of affairs, and predict the future with some certitude. As part of a liberal education, kinesiology students develop a cultural awareness that spans time and a critical sensitivity to human dilemmas through the ages. In the words of Spears and Swanson (1988), authors of a leading history text in the field, we should study history "to enrich our understanding of our civilization, our nation, and our world, . . . and to understand the historical background of today's problems" (p. 8).

The history of physical activity is as long and as varied as the history of mankind. To attempt to study all movement forms, all influential individuals and every cultural institution and practice that has affected the evolution of movement would be unreasonable in the time and context of a college curriculum. Consequently, each contemporary kinesiology program tends to select aspects of the history of human movement that reflect its specific mission while at the same time promoting certain educational objectives.

The first goal of the history portion of kinesiology is to learn how to investigate and interpret history. The purpose of liberal education is to create independent learners, those who have been empowered to continue acquiring knowledge and gaining understanding long beyond the years of formal education. Knowing how to frame meaningful questions, where to look for answers, and how to interpret evidence leading to plausible interpretations are the *skills of historical inquiry* necessary for ongoing independent learning.

In studying the history of kinesiology, the second goal is to trace the impact of cultural attitudes, practices and key individuals on the study of human movement in higher education. A starting point in this endeavor is the appreciation of our western heritage, which entails more than a passing acquaintance with ancient Greek society. From these roots emerged a nexus of ideas that have influenced the study of human movement for two millennia, often in conflicting ways. In more recent times, sportive physical activity emerged to dominate scholarship in physical education in higher education. The confluence of socio-cultural forces that produced, and have continued to shape, modern sporting practice are pre-conditions of the emergence of sport history in higher education.

The third goal in studying the history of human movement is to describe *the forces that have affected the study of human movement in higher education*. One of the features that distinguishes kinesiology in the present from physical education of the past is the inclusion of supportive and expressive forms of human movement in current curricula. Looking back to the emergence of an emphasis upon sportive movement in physical education and the more recent developments that have reintroduced alternative forms of movement into contemporary kinesiology, provides context for understanding this emerging field of study.

The aim of this chapter is to describe:

▶ the historical inquiry skills necessary in kinesiology.

▶ the cultural attitudes and practices, the individuals, and events that have most influenced the study of human movement in higher education through the ages.

▶ the modern history of emergence of a broad base of human movement studies in higher education.

Asking the right questions is as critical in historical investigation as it is in philosophical inquiry or scientific research. Spears and Swanson (1988) recommended that students of sport history keep three criteria in mind when asking questions:

*1) Does evidence exist that permits me to answer the question? 2) Does evidence exist that shows me how to place the question and answer in the proper social, economic and political contexts? and 3) What will I know after I have answered the question? Is it significant? (p.7)*

Care should be taken not only in formulating meaningful, accessible questions but also in interpreting historical data that might lead to answers. A safeguard against slipshod scholarship is rigorous research. This involves delving into as many sources of primary evidence as can be found, consisting of indisputable firsthand information that may illuminate the question. If primary sources cannot be located, reliable, carefully interpreted, secondary sources derived from firsthand evidence can provide supplementary information. Other attributes necessary for historical inquiry are curiosity, rigor, and research vigor, and the philosophical tools of deductive and inductive logic. Much like a detective (Winks, 1968), the scholar bent on solving a historical mystery unearths all the available evidence, scrutinizes it for logical contradictions, and makes supportable inferences when data are not available, to reach a plausible verdict. If a conclusion is to be acceptable, researchers have to avoid imposing personal values and current cultural standards upon events of the past. Ethnocentric judgments are easy to make in the face of actions and values that seem bigoted or ignorant by today's standards. To dismiss the context of history, however, is to fail to understand the nature of historical research and inquiry.

An alternative recourse for neophyte historians seeking answers to the puzzles of the past is to seek out the wisdom that has been accumulated in the field. Historians already have collected, collated, and classified the bulk of the information that might be useful to kinesiology students today — mostly in the latter part of the 20th century, although recognition of the importance of historical understanding existed a hundred years ago. Edward Hartwell, president of the American Association for the Advancement of Physical Education (AAAPE) from 1891–1892, was a proponent of placing the physiology of exercise and health in a historical context (Hartwell, 1886, 1899). Luther Gulick, (1890) president of the AAAPE from 1903 to 1907, espoused the value of historical research and scholarship as an integral part of the newly emerging profession of physical education.

In the first third of the 20th century, a small group of individuals was writing about the historical value of studying sports and the historical development of sports themselves. Not until 1937, however, did Seward Staley, a professor of physical education at the University of Illinois, suggest that a course in the history of sport should be a part of physical educators' professional preparation. As sport history gradually found a foothold in the curriculum, it became a topic of concern to professional associations. In 1960, Marvin Eyler began efforts to establish a section devoted to sport history within the College Physical Education Association (CPEA). In 1962, a section for sport history became a reality within the CPEA. It was a public forum and a disseminating agent of new ideas in sport history.

The 1970s were a time of considerable growth in interest and organization. In 1971, the Big Ten Symposium on the History of Physical Education and Sport was held at the Ohio State University. In 1972, the North American Society for Sport History (NASSH) was founded, and Eyler was named its first president. Since 1970, associations for the historical study of sport have emerged in 10 countries and, subsequently, the International Association for the History of Physical Education and Sport was founded in 1971. The journals of these associations — the *Journal of Sport History*, established in 1974, and the *British Journal of Sports History*, established a decade later — are primary sources of historical information. Articles pertaining to the history of sport also can be found in the *Research Quarterly for Exercise and Sport*, the *American Historical Review*, the *Journal of American History*, the *Journal of Social History*, the *Journal of American Studies*, and *Isis*. The historical inquiry skills necessary for successful library and archive research include:

▶ facility with library organization and computer searching.

▶ judicious selection of pertinent sources.

▶ discrimination between evidence of varying quality.

▶ discernment of applicability of resource content.

▶ accurate and complete referencing when reporting findings.

## PAST INFLUENCES ON THE STUDY OF HUMAN MOVEMENT IN HIGHER EDUCATION

Understanding how the study of human movement has evolved in higher education involves analyzing the attitudes and practices that existed at the time of conception of the first western university. Those first programs, based on prevailing notions of what constituted education, formed the basis of college curricula. Any attempt to reform physical education/kinesiology since that time has been premised upon this heritage. The accumulated wisdom of the ancient world fundamentally influenced modern higher education. Understanding the inheritance of the modern world of higher education from the ancient world is one of the important stanchions of historical knowledge in kinesiology.

Physical activity has been a significant phenomenon throughout the history of humankind, for it is linked to the unchangeable, neurophysiological nature of human existence. In *Sports and Games in the Ancient World*, Olivova (1984) elaborated upon the culturally specific nature of physical activities in the ancient world:

## EARLY INFLUENCES

*They were influenced by the character and structure of society. They were a significant cultural phenomenon, reflecting contemporary ideas about the world, and moral and aesthetic norms, the degree of social differentiation, and the political evolution of society. All these factors determined the many and changing forms of these activities at different moments in history. (p. 9)*

At the earliest moments in history, people learned to use their physical abilities to engage in the useful activities of gathering food, hunting, and doing all forms of physical labor necessary for their survival. When society progressed beyond the stage of a hunting economy, hunting and fighting became distinct activities, each of which required training and preparation in the form of game simulation for the young. Rhythmic movement evolved at festivals and communal dances, which generally combined the features of ritualistic natural religion and ecstatic dancing, often to a trancelike state. Olivova (1984) noted the relevance of understanding these early movement forms for appreciating movement today:

*In these communal dances movement assumed a wide variety of forms, presenting in embryo the many activities that were later, after specific development, to form separate disciplines, ranging from dance itself to drama. (p. 14)*

Festivals featured trials of strength and combative ability. They were an occasion for tribal leaders to exercise their powers and to demonstrate their prowess in front of spectators, who gradually were appearing on the scene. Simple forms of sporting contest in pastoral and agricultural societies have been identified through ethnographic evidence as running races, wrestling, boxing, shoot contests, fencing with various weapons, jumping, throwing, swimming, rowing, riding animals, chariot racing, and ball games. The latest archaeological evidence has revealed that these activities were especially popular in the foothills of the mountains of the Near East, in the ancient societies of Mesopotamia flourishing between the Tigris and the Euphrates, in ancient Egypt, and around the Mediterranean, particularly on the island of Crete. Much of modern sport has its antecedents in the activities of these ancient civilizations. "Modern sport evolved as part of the culture of Europe, but the foundations of this culture had been crystallizing for thousands of years in the context of the ancient civilizations" (Olivova, 1984, p. 9).

## The Greek Influence

The civilization of Greece, which absorbed elements from all of these sources to form its own culture, is of particular importance to modern western experience. The cultural values and physical practices of the ancient Greek civilization have influenced contemporary thought and practice immeasurably.

*From the sixth to the fourth centuries B.C. in particular, there appeared to be a balance among all of one's daily activities, and sport appeared to play a greater role in normal life than in any other society to this point. (Howell and Howell, p. 29)*

The Greek civilization dates back to about 1700 B.C., when the Achaeans (known as the Mycenaean culture) dominated in Greece. By the 9th century B.C., the classical Greeks (Hellenic culture) began to emerge in the form of city states such as Corinth, Athens, and Sparta. Their survival and security depended upon their military prowess, so warlike, patriotic people such as the Spartans, characterized as being disciplined, brave, and obedient, were able to thrive in this climate. The Athenian Greeks, however, are most frequently cited as role models for today in many of their customs and attitudes. During the process of establishing a secure city-state, the Athenians were aggressive and territorial, not unlike the Spartans. Through exercise of their intellectual energy, however, they crafted a culture that emphasized a balanced lifestyle between wisdom and exercise, civic responsibility and personal development, military readiness and "the good life."

This concept of balance found its expression in physical activity in the everyday life of the community. Gymnasia and palaestrae (wrestling schools) were built throughout the city, and these gave impetus to athletic festivals. The buildings were multipurpose areas that often included recreation rooms and lounging rooms for poets, philosophers, and musicians. They provided "the citizens a place to meet and talk, to exercise, and to perform various physical activities" (Howell & Howell, 1988, p. 30).

Typical of the harmony between the physical and intellectual dimensions of cultural life in Athens was that individuals famously associated with philosophy also were athletically inclined. Aristotle often taught at the Lyceum, and Plato might be found not only teaching at the Academy but also wrestling (in the Isthmian Games), a sport that Pericles also favored. Three of the four national (Panhellenic) games — the Isthmian, the Pythian, and the Nemean festivals — were established in the early part of the 6th century. The fourth of these Panhellenic Games had been held many times already at the site of the religious sanctuary of Olympia, where the confluence of the rivers Alpheius and Clideus formed a natural alluvial plain. The official olympic register dates back to 776 B. C., when Corebus of Elis, the victor in a running race, had his name inscribed in perpetuity, but evidence indicates that unrecorded games preceded that date.

The athletic emphasis at these games was upon events such as foot racing, the pentathlon (which consisted of jumping, discus, javelin, a one-stage foot race, and wrestling), heavy events (such as boxing, wrestling and pankratian, which combined boxing and wrestling into a rough-and-tumble event) and chariot racing (particularly at Olympia, which had a reputation for horse breeding). All the games featured a balance between athletics, music, poetry, and drama. These games prompted balance in another way, too: by fostering political democracy. Through competition in the Panhellenic Games, citizen-athletes could improve their upward mobility. As James Thompson (1988) observed, "Solon's legislation, in a sense, democratized athletics in Athens since the opportunity to compete in the national festivals became less exclusively the privilege of the elite class" (p. 184).

Competitive activity was complemented by the rhythm, harmony, and music of dance that permeated the lives of the Athenians: "They danced in the temples, the woods, the fields. Every event of interest to the family, every birth, every marriage, every death, was the occasion of a dance." (Vuillier, 1898, p.7). Through their emphases upon beauty and goodness (kalos kagathos), all-around excellence (arete), and harmony, the Greeks gave the physical dimension:

*. . . a respectability that it has never since achieved. They accorded the body equal dignity with the mind. They associated sport with philosophy, music, literature, painting, and particularly with sculpture. They gave to all future civilizations important aesthetic ideals and the ideals of harmonized balance of mind and body, of body symmetry, and of bodily beauty in repose and in action. To these contributions may be added educational gymnastics, the competitive sports of track and field, the classic dance, and the Olympic Games. (Van Dalen & Bennett, 1971, p. 47)*

In the later years of the Greek civilization, after the Persian wars, as Athens became a major industrial and commercial center, its citizens became more oriented toward personal success than toward civic service. The emphasis of education changed from civic and physical training to the life of the mind. Physical activity became the realm of the paid professional, to the detriment of the principles of moderation and all-around physical development.

## The Roman Age

The Greek orientation carried into the Roman Age, 500 B. C. to 476 A.D. The early Romans were a conservative people who sought utility in their actions. Their emphasis on the physical centered on strength and hardiness, in contrast to the holistic approach of the Greeks of Periclean Athens, who in addition valued beauty and grace. In many ways, the Roman system of military training for international dominance resembled that of Sparta, although training was given at home, not in state-run military barracks.

As the Roman civilization expanded, contact with the outside world through conquest made the Romans realize the value of intellectual education. Consequently, schools were founded for the ruling and commercial groups. Roman education paid scant attention to physical components, although the emperors promoted games and festivals to occupy and appease Roman subjects. In general, the participatory, holistic emphasis of the "golden age" of Greece was replaced by professionalized, often brutal, spectator-oriented contests. After the Roman conquest of Greece, even the Panhellenic games, changed from events of grace and beauty to games characterized by brutality, professionalism, and corruption.

Throughout the later years of the Greek empire and the entire Roman era, intellectuals from various walks of life looked back admiringly, even wistfully, at the ways in which the Athenian Greeks connected their physical existence with all aspects of their cultural life. As an example, Horace, the "Roman Pindar," was a respected poet who sought to encourage physical fitness among youth in the late first century B. C. by vigorously endorsing a Greek athletic program in the context of Roman education (Scanlon, 1984, p. 163). And Galen of Pergamon (A. D. 129–post-210), personal physician to Emperor Marcus Aurelius and one of the great figures in the history of medicine, was caustically critical of the artificial training methods and excesses of professional athletics which departed from the Greek principle of the golden mean. He strongly supported a return to the natural movements provided through rowing, jumping, fencing, carrying weights, throwing the javelin, and riding on horseback, and particularly ball games that exercised the whole body in a natural way. He preferred these activities for reasons of health and because the balanced program of physical training the Athenian Greeks developed still had philosophical appeal and social benefits (Scarborough, 1985, p. 171).

After the fall of the Roman empire in 476 A. D., the Teutonic tribes ushered in the Dark Ages of civilization. Throughout this period and until modern times, several enduring themes of great importance to the study of human movement in higher education have been intertwined with western society's evolving belief systems and cultural institutions. Understanding these themes is the key to appreciating the legacy of human movement. The central theme underlying cultural and educational practice is that the intellectual orientation of western culture toward the study of human movement and the body emanates from two conflicting approaches to "things physical" generated by Greek culture. The naturalistic concept of balance and integration (associated with Periclean anthropology and education in Athens) has vied for popular acceptance through the ages with the notion of one's physical being as subservient to one's intellectual processes (the concept of a "learning mind and a behaving body" (Metheny, 1965, p. 5).

Even though Plato was an advocate of healthful living and exemplified a balance of intellectual and physical vigor in his own life, he is credited as the progenitor of metaphysical dualism. Plato was a paradox in that he subscribed to two streams of philosophical thought: "One is a kind of supernaturalism, consistent with his idealistic philosophy and with the Orphic religion; the other is a kind of naturalism consistent with his realistic philosophy and with the traditional Greek religion" (Feibleman, p. 67).

The role and status of kinesiology today, and of physical education in the past, in the process of higher education has been determined culturally by how this dilemma of the relationship between body and mind has been resolved. Landmarks in the history of physical education are monuments to cultural changes in this mentality. Major changes in the cultural history of the study of movement have been precipitated by reversal of the hierarchical order of mind and body. For instance, the shift from the highly commercialized, professionalized, spectator sports scene of third and fourth century Graeco-Roman culture to the ascetic anti-play spirit of medieval culture was the result of the soul's reversing hierarchical position with the body.

Figure 7.1 illustrates the effects of this central theme, or idea, about human movement on cultural practices through the ages. Cultural attitudes and practices are not constant. They change in relation to a dominant cultural mentality. This affects the nature of cultural practices including education, religion, medicine, and sport, as well as the individual's intellectual orientation and cultural behavior. Pitirim

## ENDURING THEMES

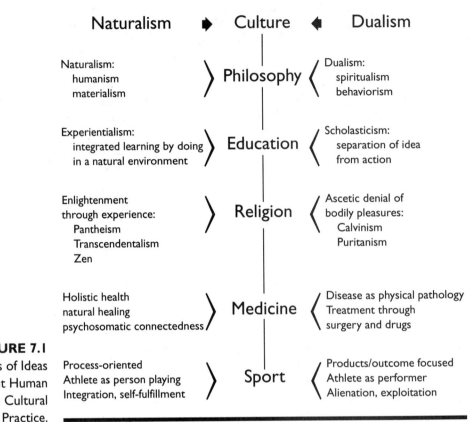

Naturalism   ⬧ Culture ◀ Dualism

Naturalism:
  humanism
  materialism   ⟩ **Philosophy** ⟨   Dualism:
    spiritualism
    behaviorism

Experientialism:
  integrated learning by doing ⟩ **Education** ⟨ Scholasticism:
  in a natural environment     separation of idea
    from action

Enlightenment
through experience:   ⟩ **Religion** ⟨ Ascetic denial of
  Pantheism   bodily pleasures:
  Transcendentalism     Calvinism
  Zen     Puritanism

Holistic health
natural healing ⟩ **Medicine** ⟨ Disease as physical pathology
psychosomatic connectedness   Treatment through
    surgery and drugs

Process-oriented
Athlete as person playing ⟩ **Sport** ⟨ Products/outcome focused
Integration, self-fulfillment   Athlete as performer
    Alienation, exploitation

**FIGURE 7.1**

Historical Effects of Ideas About Human Movement on Cultural Practice.

Sorokin (1957), a distinguished Harvard sociologist, suggested that the history of western culture is one of flux between the extremes of materialism and spiritualism. Only rarely are these extremes confluent, at which times the materialistic and spiritualistic components of the cultural mentality converge to create a unified synthesis, an emphasis upon "the whole person." Sorokin's study neatly profiled the history of physical education by demonstrating that the cultural mentality of the whole person — the concept of a balanced program of physical and intellectual education — reigned supreme only in Greece during the fifth century B. C. and again during the Renaissance period. (Sorokin, 1957, pp. 240–214).

The figure illustrates how cultural practices have responded to the dominant cultural mentality during the brief (three centuries) of balanced emphasis upon the whole person, designated *naturalism*, and throughout the other two millennia of *dualism*. Because the cultural practices and institutions of philosophy, education, religion, medicine, and sport are indicators of how the dominant cultural mentality may affect society as a whole, each is discussed briefly here.

A naturalistic *philosophy* places people at the center of their universe, emphasizes being and becoming, and involves physical existence as an integral part of that humanistic process. Dualism subdivides people into discrete components allowing the placement of hierarchical value upon one component (e.g., mind) over another (e.g., matter).

This leads to an *educational process* in which one's physical being is a peripheral consideration. This emphasis in higher education upon ideas at the expense of action is known as *scholasticism*. If physical activity has any place in a university premised upon the principle of scholasticism, it is in keeping the body healthy and out of mischief so it may help the mind to be more alert and receptive to the intellectual process. Rarely have modern western universities digressed from this model of scholasticism to emphasize learning through doing, the experiential process, and a holistic approach to education.

Western *religion* has tended to separate body from soul to create *asceticism*, self-denial based upon the premise that indulgence in physical pleasure may distract from spiritual devotion, at the least, and might even be sinful. Long periods of history have been dominated by this religious mentality, most notably during the ascendancy of the early Christian church and after the Reformation, in the 16th century, when Lutheranism, Calvinism, and later, Puritanism became popular. The church generally has decried play and other pursuits of the flesh except when they serve to keep the hands from mischief and maintain the body as "the temple of the Lord." Religion based on naturalism never has found great popularity in the western tradition, although gaining enlightenment through physical experience is a central feature of many eastern religions, most notably Zen Buddhism. In the West, the naturalistic philosophy of Rousseau, transcendentalism as proposed by Emerson, and the pantheistic beliefs of Wordsworth and Thoreau are examples of belief systems since the Enlightenment that place physical sensation at the center of spiritual experience.

In more modern times, many individuals have had spiritual ("peak") experiences in and through their physical activities (Ravizza, 1977), and others claim that sport is a form of natural religion (Novak, 1976).

With few exceptions, the history of western *medicine* has been based on a dualistic tradition of treating the human body for disease and injury, rather than of healing the whole person. In contrast, throughout the long tradition of eastern medicine, the integrity of the human organism and the forces of healing beyond the treatment of symptoms of disease have been important. The western approach has gravitated toward localized surgery and the prescription of artificially synthesized chemicals to ease the pain and treat the ailment. Eastern methods more typically are directed to the body's healing forces (e.g., chi force), the interconnectedness of mind and body (e.g., acupuncture) and nature's healing power (e.g., herbal medicine).

The western tradition also has been dualistic within the physical realm of *play*, *games*, and *sport*. The dualism in sport becomes apparent when the athlete becomes performer first and person second, when the extrinsic product (winning) takes overwhelming priority over the intrinsic process (playing), and when the human body becomes an object of manipulation and exploitation.

In stark contrast to the dualistic otherworldliness that had characterized medieval life, the *Renaissance* reveled in the quality of being, encouraged the exercise of worldly talents, and emphasized harmonious development of the whole personality. Beginning in Italy in the 14th century with the works of scholars such as Petrarch, this humanistic spirit rapidly spread throughout Europe, stimulating progress in all fields of endeavor and reconstructing social and educational values. Van Dalen and Bennett (1971) noted that, "The new spirit of intellectual inquiry undermined the structure of scholasticism" (p. 123).

Although the holistic, humanistic focus on things human rather than things divine did not override the dualistic perception of the mind and body as separate frontiers, it did lead to general acceptance of the classical ideal of "the sound mind in the sound body." The paintings of Leonardo da Vinci, based on the study of human anatomy, are indicative that the human form and the beauty of the human body in motion became important in the fine arts. Popular vernacular writings about healthy physical development and cultivating beauty in and through one's physical being led to an emphasis in education upon daily exercise, childhood games, a balanced diet, and good health. At all levels of the educational process, humanists encouraged their students to think freely but to emulate classical role models, to develop their individual aptitudes but to promote balance and harmony within their own lifestyles. The physical dimension was an intrinsic feature of the humanistic education of the early Renaissance.

As the Renaissance spread to Northern Europe, its character changed from humanistic emphasis upon the wisdom of the classics to incorporate realism, culminating in a quest for knowledge through scientific inquiry. Descartes, Copernicus and Galileo were among the scholars who, through observation and experimentation, challenged the traditional understandings of the world and people's place in it. These realists advocated using the human senses as a conduit to comprehension, which naturally brought attention to the body. Van Dalen and Bennett (1971) described how the advent of realism increased scholarly interest in the human body, its capacities, and its movement. "Curiosity about the physiological laws governing the body and the mind opened the pedagogical door wider for the establishment of an improved physical education" (p. 173). Ever since the Renaissance period, the scientific logic and methodology of realism and the humanistic emphasis upon classical knowledge have pervaded higher education.

The history of the study of human movement in higher education is inextricably interwoven with the cultural fabric of the age. Yet, the actions of many early pioneers transcend their cultural context and continue to have an impact today.

During the *17th century* most western nations were caught in a struggle between reason and authority, liberty and despotism, the Reformation and the coming Age of Enlightenment. The evolution of political democracy during this period found its expression in education through the ideas of scholars such as John Locke (1632–1704). He was instrumental in seeking solutions to the problems of his time, many of which have continued to influence educational thought today. His strong belief in religious tolerance and the political rights of people have been woven into the fabric of modern education. The disciplinarianism of the age is evident in his philosophy that children are empty vessels to be filled with knowledge, that desirable behavior patterns should be practiced and enforced continually, and that a well disciplined character can be achieved only through a sound mind and a sound body. He advocated open air and exercise to toughen bodies and build resistance but discouraged play and recreational amusement. Vestiges of Locke's educational philosophy are evident in the practice and study of physical activity throughout the education system today.

The *18th century* heralded the Age of Enlightenment, a period of transition to modern political, social, religious, and educational ideas. In France, Jean Jacques Rousseau (1712–1778) laid the foundation for an egalitarian system of education by attacking the inequality of people. Like John Locke, he condemned the education of children as though they were little adults, preferring instead to allow them to develop naturally. The form of naturalism he described in Emile (Rousseau, 1911) echoed earlier Greek attitudes in that it made no distinction between the education of the mind and the body.

In Germany, Johann Friedrich Gutsmuths (1749–1839) combined the naturalism of Rousseau, the medically based concern for health of John Locke, and Renaissance realism into a program of physical education that he described in *Gymnastics for the Young* (Gutsmuths, 1800), and instituted at the Salzmann school. The main goal of this program was good health through gymnastic exercises based on knowledge of physiology and medicine. He reasoned that, because of the nature of the maturation process, growth and development of the body should be the initial emphasis of education. In contrast to the austere approach of scholars influenced by the moralism of the Restoration, Gutsmuths designed exercises that were enjoyable and encouraged women to engage in light exercises. In his recognition of the importance of the scientific bases of exercise, his emphasis upon naturalism in content, method and environment (he encouraged the use of fields and school-yards when suitable buildings were not available), and in his willing-ness to countenance women's need of exercise, Gutsmuths laid the foundation for much philosophy and practice today.

The *19th century* was generally a time of patriotic pride and indus-trial modernization. In America and France, successful revolutions gave rise to nationalistic and liberal movements. The period was marked by pride in military power, claims of racial superiority, and concern for national history and literature. Education became accepted as an effec-tive means of ensuring the welfare and progress of the nation. The surge in democracy meant that previously disenfranchised groups became empowered and that education no longer was a privilege of the elite classes and selected religious groups. This nationalistic philosophy permeated physical education practices in Europe and America.

In Germany, Friedrich Jahn (1778–1852) was hailed as an expo-nent of German unity and a defender of the commoner. He founded the Turner societies, which became popular in parts of America (e.g., Philadelphia) when they were brought into the country by German immigrants. The methods he espoused in gymnastics were based on the faith that high standards of physical proficiency were a key to national regeneration. His gymnastics system was not merely a tool for develop-ing physical well being but also a means of achieving political goals through development of a sturdy citizenry with a strong love of homeland.

In Sweden, Per Henrik Ling (1776–1839) adopted a philosophy of exercise similar to Jahn's. In founding Swedish gymnastics, he joined forces with philosophers, poets, and soldiers to develop and rebuild the prestige and honor of Sweden. With the nationalistic purpose of raising physical standards of the army, Ling's program emphasized power, alacrity of action, and ability to endure strain. He also designed pro-grams of medical gymnastics that would restore health through exer-cise. In so doing, he set the tone for later developments in the United States in the areas of supportive movement such as proactive health care and the development of physical therapy and other forms of exercise therapy treatments.

Using gymnastic exercise to create a sense of nationalism throughout Europe (e.g., Frans Nachtegall, 1777–1847, in Denmark) initiated the trend of intertwining gymnastic exercise and other forms of physical activity (most notably, sport) with politics. To be sure, the rulers of some earlier civilizations, such as the Roman Empire, had tried to keep bread on the table and sport in the stadia of their citizenry ("bread and circuses") to keep the proletariat content and to divert their energies from insurgence. These European initiatives, however, were not systems of exercise imposed upon the proletariat by a ruling class but, rather, nationalistic programs of exercise freely chosen by the citizens of democracies. The actions of Jahn and Ling, in particular, who designed gymnastic systems that would become most popular in the United States, set a precedent for the political overtones in future American programs of exercise and sport.

To explain the history of physical activity and sport, and their study, in the United States, Spears and Swanson (1988) explicated the following themes:

## MODERN AMERICAN THEMES

*The expectations of "the good life" for every citizen, the diversity in which American culture is grounded, the perceived values that govern daily living, social organization, the intermixing of technology and urbanization, and the conceptualization of today's sport and physical education. (p. 13)*

The pursuit of happiness, or *the good life* is the "inalienable right" that framers of the U. S. Declaration of Independence premised upon the other two rights: "life and liberty." In the more than 200 years since the 1776 signing, Americans have exercised their life and liberty to pursue their own ideals of happiness. Beyond the necessities of life, such as financial security, lie an array of qualities of existence that many Americans have chosen to make their priorities and that directly impinge on kinesiology. For example, excellent health through exercise and dieting, recreational activities during leisure time, and watching and playing sports have gathered momentum as generally accepted features of "the good life" ever since the first colonists arrived on American shores.

## The Good Life

These colonists, and later immigrants, contributed to the *diversity* of cultural values and physical practices of "the melting pot" of the United States. During the *colonial period* (1607–1790), settlers brought their distinctive ethnic traditions and physical pastimes to the areas in which they congregated. Examples of the regional flavor of games and sports during this period were the preference of the Dutch colonists in New York for bowling, skating, and hunting; the sports of Britain finding a home in Virginia; and the noticeable lack of playful physical activities in New England as a result of the restrictive Puritan influence.

## Diversity

During the *national period*, after the revolution against British rule, the amusements and sports of these immigrants had to be adapted not only to the many different living patterns in America but also to the emerging sense of nationalism sweeping across the nation. Eventually, groups that had been narrowly ethnic in focus became assimilated into mainstream culture or slipped into decline. For example, the Turner method met with opposition from communities until 1880, when the Turners began to teach in English instead of German and became instrumental in promoting their brand of gymnastics not only in the Turnvereine but also in the schools of the larger community that surrounded them. Games and sports brought from the immigrants' more than 50 countries of origin were adapted to suit American ways (e.g., American football). The search for national identity found expression through the invention of popular sports including basketball (1892) and volleyball (1895) and through debate over what should constitute an American system of exercise.

## Values

The pursuit of happiness and the cultural values of immigrants from various ethnic backgrounds historically have coalesced to create a system of *values* that guides and influences Americans' daily work lives and play habits. The early influence of the New England Puritans, who perceived play to be unrighteous, affected when and how people might participate in sport. The virility of this belief system led to frequent attacks on play. "Attacks were directed at almost every form of amusement: dancing for its carnality; rough-and-tumble ball games for their violence; maypoles for their paganism; and sports in general because they were often played on the Sabbath" (Sage, 1990, p. 90).

As the nation has gradually become secularized, laws restricting sportive behavior on Sundays and taboos on who might play (e.g., women) have been liberalized. Even during the latter part of the 18th century, people enjoyed activities such as horse racing, cock fighting, running races, and wrestling, often in defiance of local laws. Many games, such as bowling, billiards, darts, horseshoes and card games, grew up around the taverns that often were the secular social centers of society. Values varied from region to region, and from individual to individual, so differences have continued to exist concerning topics such as whether people should play on the Sabbath, how much brutality is acceptable in sport, and whether animals should compete in "blood sports" (e.g., cock fighting). Nevertheless, the general increase in leisure time, discretionary income, and emphasis on healthful living, particularly since the Industrial Revolution began in the 19th century, have tended to promote participation in physical pastimes.

The social organization of American society historically has dictated who might have access to which sportive opportunities. Throughout American history, a combination of ideology associated with sporting practice and social stratification have affected sportive and educative human movement. The ethos and practice of many of the games imported from Britain had been the sole dominion of a privileged, wealthy minority. Although some games (such as soccer) had a more egalitarian background, other games (such as croquet, rugby, cricket, track and field, and rowing), which attracted a large following in 19th-century America, had been the dominion of the upper class in English public schools.

The ideology that had permeated these activities in England took root in American soil. In particular, the ideology of *amateurism* (which had been popular with a privileged minority of people who did not need to be reimbursed for their performance) and the cult of *masculinity* (based on the prescription of physical activities to develop manly virtues in the all-male public school environment) continued to affect sporting practice in the United States. In the latter part of the 19th century, athletic clubs that limited their membership to upper-class gentlemen-amateurs grew up in England and then in the United States, and American universities modeled themselves after the British prototype amateur. Similarly, George Sage (1990) observed that the cult of manliness "became widely pervasive in the upper and middle classes and rapidly trickled down to working class social life" (p. 98). M. L. Adelman (1986) explained this phenomenon.

*The frequency with which writers began to assert that sport could serve as a means of promoting manliness was in direct response to both the impact of modernization on urban society and the role of modernization in redefining the masculine role and creating a new middle class view of proper sexual behavior. (p. 283)*

The early organization of American society contributed its own series of restrictions to the access and conduct of games and sport. Although the Declaration of Independence claimed that "all men are created equal" with certain inalienable rights, the reality of the situation was that, "in spite of the founders' high ideals and the optimistic expectations of the settlers and immigrants, the realities of economic and social life have led to social classes in this country" (Spears & Swanson, 1988, p. 11). The colonist conquests of native American Indians, the subsequent practice of slavery in the southern states, and the continuing subjugation of women created disenfranchised classes of people who participated in their own activities but who did not have access to public education and the sports establishment until relatively recently in American history.

Social stratification, based on gender, race, wealth, and age, have radically affected the history of the study of human movement in higher education. For example, because of gender role expectations, women have had limited access to forms of movement that require extreme vigor, physical contact and combative strength and to higher education throughout much of American history. Catherine Beecher was ahead of her time when she founded the Hartford Female Seminary in 1828, because women were not admitted routinely to universities nationwide for another century. Although YWCAs offered young women the opportunity to participate in light exercises and swimming as long ago as the latter part of the 19th century, women did not win legal recognition of their equality of opportunity in sport until passage of Title IX of the Educational Amendments Act of 1972.

## Technology/ Urbanization

The roots of America's sporting heritage lie in horse racing, fox hunting, and other colonial pastimes, but not until the agrarian and frontier economy gave way to industrialization and urbanization in the mid-19th century did modern sport began to emerge. The congregation in cities of masses of immigrants and workers who left their farms to seek riches in the factories signaled a change from the rustic pleasures of hunting and fishing to commercialized entertainment and spectator sports. The character of life changed to make sport an attractive outlet for citizens with more money, more surplus energy than existed after a day of laboring in the fields, more regular hours with predictable free time for leisure activities, and greater need to prove their physical prowess in a more sanitized, safe, living environment. The combination of urbanization, industrialization, and new technology created rapid growth in sport so that:

*By 1900 sport had attained an unprecedented prominence in the daily lives of millions of Americans, and this remarkable development had been achieved in great part through the steamboat, the railroad, the telegraph, the penny press, the electric light, the streetcar, the camera, the bicycle, the automobile, and the mass production of sporting goods. (Betts, 1953, p. 232)*

The very character of sports as we know and study them today was shaped by the progress and practices of this period. Some of the activities that had been popular before 1850, such as cricket and fencing, fell from favor while others, such as rowing, running, prize fighting, and horse racing, were the early beneficiaries of the "Yankee ingenuity" of the times. Early forms of mass transportation, such as steamboats were superseded by an elaborate railroad network that served as a common carrier of sport *spectators*. Developments in transportation, which later would include the bicycle and the automobile, soon were matched by breakthroughs in *communication technology* that presaged the role of the *media* as a purveyor of sports to the general public. As examples: invention of the telegraph, in 1844, led to expansion of the sporting news and extensive betting on events; completion of the Atlantic cable in 1866 promoted international communications; and the forerunner of the modern radio, the wireless, was first used to cover the yacht races of 1899. An important feature of modern sport is *standardization* of rules, and of equipment. Mass production methods of manufacturing (e.g., baseball equipment by A. G. Spalding and Brothers) brought parity to the playing field, where the size of the bat and the dimensions of the ball previously had been the defining features of performance. Sport became commercialized as entrepreneurs developing new technology and retail conglomerates selling uniforms and equipment (such as Macy's of New York and Sears, Roebuck and Company) gained a vested interest in the continuing success of evolving sports. Thomas Edison's invention of the light bulb in 1879 inaugurated a whole new era of social and sporting life in the cities, permitting players and spectators to indulge in their interests beyond normal daylight working hours. The character of sport changed during this period to gain *mass appeal*, so that, by 1890, "a decade of electrification, paralleling improvements in transportation and communications, had elevated and purified the atmosphere of sport" (Betts, 1953, p. 240). Betts cited prize fighting as one example of a sport that underwent a metamorphosis during this period. "The saloon brawls of pugilists in the 1850s and 1860s were gradually abandoned for the organized matches of the 1880s and 1890s" (p. 240). Technological developments in the latter half of the 19th century and beyond transformed the social habits of the western world and, in so doing, revolutionized modern sport.

## Conceptualization of Today's Sport

The final theme affecting the evolution of modern sport in America is "the changing conceptualization and justification of sport and physical education" (Spears & Swanson, 1988, p. 13). Modern sport has assumed a major role in popular culture and American society. It has become intertwined with other major social institutions such as politics, economics, education, and mass media. It continues to play a role in the lives of most of the American public, as players and spectators, in the forms of intensive participation and daily dialogue. Through analysis of the history of sport in the United States several themes emerge to explain its conceptual popularity:

1. Far removed from the hardships early colonists and frontiersmen endured, the physical challenge of daily existence has declined gradually in the time since the agrarian, industrial-manufacturing, and information eras of the nation's history. Sport has taken an equal but opposite growth pattern, becoming, by nature and through choice, more risk-oriented and vigorous throughout its evolution.

2. Increasing anonymity and alienation accompany industrialization, urbanization, and city life. As the extended family, which provided emotional sustenance in rural settings, was broken up by the mobility and transience of modern existence, sport offered an alternative form of communal identification and mutual endeavor.

3. The perceived potential for character building in and through sport gave impetus to the playground movements in many cities, the growth of the "Y's," the popularity of the Turner movement, and the evolution of muscular Christianity (which spawned such evangelical groups as Athletes in Action). This positive effect upon personality was one of the reasons given for integrating sports programs into public education, for public and private sponsorship of sports, and for advertising through sports.

Public perception of the physical, social and moral value of sports has led to an exponential growth pattern, particularly since the middle of the 19th century.

Historical justification of the form growth has taken entails consideration of the popularity of the professional sports model and the process of integrating sport into the nation's educational system. Professional and intercollegiate sports, have been the focal point of the historical popularity of sport. Industrialization provided the financial wherewithal; urbanization created the spectator potential; and technology contributed standardization, media focus, and equipment. The Civil War pointed up the nation's deficient manpower and gave impetus to leagues of professional athletes and athletic clubs. Baseball was one of the first games to be professionalized. The Cincinnati Red Stockings team was formed in 1869, followed by teams in Philadelphia, Boston, and other cities. Professional sport might have foundered at this early stage if not for the efforts of William Hulbert and A. G. Spalding to deliver baseball from the gambling and corruption that surrounded the game at first.

College sports seemed to be following a similar path toward professionalism at their outset. The first intercollegiate contest, a crew race between Harvard and Yale in 1852, was sponsored by a railroad company that transported both teams and their spectators to Lake Win-nipesaukee and reimbursed the contestants appropriately for their efforts. As Ronald Smith (1988) stated, in *Sports and Freedom: The Rise of Big-Time College Athletics*:

*There can be no doubt that nearly every important institution of higher education in America has at some point in its history emphasized big-time intercollegiate athletics. . . . From the first contest, intercollegiate sport has been a commercial enterprise, and professionalism followed closely on its heels. (p. ix)*

Yet, the justification for including sports in the college setting was their educational benefit to the student body. This ideology had been evident in the amateurism of athletics in British universities, particularly Oxford and Cambridge, which exerted a powerful influence over the two American universities that first developed big-time athletic programs, Harvard and Yale. The tug-of-war between these competing ideologies was complicated further by the perennial questions of academic freedom, the struggle for control over athletics between faculty and students, and the hiring of the professional coach (Smith, 1988). As college sport became more entrenched in the university system, the need to establish eligibility rules, to cut back on the brutality of contests (especially football), and to create some form of interinstitutional control, led to gradual erosion of student control of student games.

In the latter part of the 19th century, faculty committees attempted to control and redirect the development of college athletics, but by the time the National Collegiate Athletic Association (NCAA) was formed in 1905, individual universities had begun to lose control of athletics to outside forces. Since that time, the NCAA and other governing bodies of college sport have tried to curb the corruption of the educational enterprise by the incursion of the professional sports model.

Throughout the 20th century, the justifications for amateur participation, including the educational benefits of sports participation, its character-building potential, and the healthy mind in a healthy body argument, have been invoked successfully to sustain athletics within the American university. Physical education basked in the reflected glow of the educational rationale for athletics by making sport a curricular centerpiece.

Contemporary analysts disagree as to whether the history of college sport may be characterized more accurately as *pluralistic* or as *hegemonic* in nature. "In the pluralistic model, sports and physical recreational activities are seen primarily as innocent, voluntary social practices that let people release tension and enjoy themselves" (Sage, 1990, p. 25). From this perspective, "Sport is often touted as an arena where `appropriate' sociocultural attitudes and beliefs are nurtured and an activity where society's collective interests are promoted and sustained" (Sage, p. 25). In contrast, from the hegemonic perspective, "Sport is viewed as promoting and supporting the social inequality endemic to capitalism. This is seen in class, gender, and race social relations and the control, production, and distribution of economic, political, and cultural power in sport" (p. 26).

## HISTORICAL SCOPE OF THE STUDY OF HUMAN MOVEMENT IN HIGHER EDUCATION

Van Dalen and Bennett (1971) suggested that "a concept of the social forces, conditions, movements, and the philosophies that have come out of the past to shape the institutions of the present day" (p. viii) is essential to appreciation of current practice. Much of the scholarship in this regard during this century has been devoted to the sportive category of human movement and its implementation in the educational system. The social forces, conditions, and philosophies that have driven most scholarly attention have been related to sport, recreation, leisure, and skill-related exercise in an educational context.

Though they are important foci within kinesiology, these facets of human movement are too narrow to adequately define the study of human movement. The study of sport traditionally has been a mainstay of physical education; however, other categories of movement have been significant to people through time. Symbolic movement has been represented through dance ever since the earliest civilizations, when expressive feelings and worship through rhythmic movement were profoundly important components of the social life of a community.

*One of the particularly significant forms of expression was that of physical movement. A special body language was created, which was not only capable of expressing and communicating ideas but of passing them on from one generation to another. (Olivova, 1984, p. 12)*

Park (1987), a leading historian in the field, decried the traditional narrowness of focus and recommended a broader conceptualization of what constitutes the history of human movement. She defined sport broadly as "a category term that includes, at the least, agonistic (characterized by the struggle of competition) athletics, vigorous recreational pursuits, and physical education, and intersects with aspects of medicine, biology, social reform, and a host of other topics" (p. 96). These intersections of physical activity with medicine, biology, and social reform comprise the historical basis of the supportive category of human movement, which is growing rapidly in popularity within kinesiology.

Earlier this century, the human movement professions veered away from this biomedical focus toward a preoccupation with sportive activity and its educative implementation in schools. Vertinsky (1991) attributed that change in emphasis to:

---

*. . . A market opportunity outside the health field, that was to influence the direction and nature of professional practice in the next half century. The possibility that physical education would develop in tandem with the biological sciences or take responsibility for popular health education faded in light of the influence of the social sciences and professional education dictates that encouraged play, games, and sports for the youth in the nation's schools (Kroll, 1971; Park, 1989). (Vertinsky, 1991, p. 75)*

---

Even so, contemporary kinesiology alliance of sportive and supportive physical activity beneath one professional umbrella had a precedent a century ago. Park (1989) traced the genesis of the "new" profession of physical education in the 1890s, "fostered in part by dramatic changes that had been occurring in the biological sciences since the early 1800s" (p. 3). It combined concern for health with education in a concerted emphasis on total physical development. Because of the potential for this intellectual union, many "social reformers, theologians, philanthropists, college presidents and educators, men and women of letters, a large number of physicians, and several biologists and psychologists subscribed to the belief that physical education might become one of the most important studies of the 20th century" (Park, 1989, p. 3).

The last two decades of the 19th century were a time of frenetic activity in the "new" profession of physical education. The Association for the Advancement of Physical Education was founded in 1885. Journal articles and books were written on the topics of health-related exercise, physical training, and athletics. The goals of the "new" profession were elucidated. As Luther Gulick (1890) pointed out, these goals were not the same as those of athletics or of any existing medical specialty, for they included (Park, 1989, p. 3):

- the establishment and maintenance of personal health.
- psychological efficiency of circulatory, respiratory, digestive, and muscular functions.
- proper development of the nervous system.
- the social, psychological, and moral development of the individual.
- improvement of the American race through the evolution of better genetic inheritance for future generations.

These goals found their expression in higher education in programs such as Harvard University's 4-year degree program in anatomy, physiology, and physical training. Established in 1891, the twin goals of this program were to prepare undergraduate students for the study of medicine and to take charge of physical training programs. The urgent societal need for physical training of professionals is attributable to the growing recognition of how the changing socioeconomic milieu of the newly industrialized cities was deleteriously affecting personal health. "Popular physiologists, doctors, and physical educators joined to advise Americans on how to adjust to modern society by using new scientific information to understand how to balance the internal needs of the body with the newly perceived demands of the environment" (Vertinsky, 1990, p. 73). Health-related fitness became equated with personal efficiency and societal regeneration. The goal of developing the fitness levels necessary to support any chosen lifestyle (supportive activity) was espoused by leaders in the field such as Dudley Sargent (1906) as "fitness for work, fitness for play, fitness for anything a man may be called upon to do" (p. 297).

As physical education evolved, school physical training and athletics became its primary concern, and health became the concern of public health departments and professional medical care. In the 20th century, medical theories, such as the germ theory of disease causation, replaced ideas of holistic prevention through physical training with a more atomistic, scientific view of the treatment of pathological conditions. As the realm of medicine slipped away from physical education, drug chemistry took the place of health and hygiene. Meanwhile, the demand for physical education teachers become a staple source of professional opportunity for university graduates, prompting many to agree with Clark Hetherington (1925) in his claim that physical education is a teaching profession, first, last, and all the time.

During the first 30 years of the 20th century, enactment of compulsory physical education laws in 22 states, the consequent shortage of teachers, and the meteoric rise in college enrollment by 75% solidified the profession's perception that teacher education is the central mission of physical education. Meanwhile, a broadening of teaching focus from education *of* the physical to education *through* the physical, led by scholars such as Dr. Thomas D. Wood of Stanford University and Clark Hetherington (who emphasized the educational process at the four levels of organic, psychomotor, character, and intellectual education), further distanced the field from the scientific study of health-related physical activity. Efforts to establish a biomedical emphasis dissipated until recent changes within kinesiology and society combined to make an applied health science approach in the human movements professions attractive and feasible.

A sense of history prevents contemporary kinesiology from drifting aimlessly into the 21st century. The trends of the past give direction to the future. The skills of historical inquiry are the basis of any investigation into past influences on the study of human movement. Early civilizations (notably ancient Greece), individual contributions (such as those of Gutsmuths and Gulick), happenings (such as the Renaissance and the Industrial Revolution) and enduring attitudes (such as ascetism and scholasticism) have helped to shape current practice. The emergence of modern sport and a national need for more teachers provided focus and a sense of purpose to the emerging field of physical education, even as such pioneers as Sargent sought to lead the new profession in a biomedical direction. The past is prologue. Efforts of the pioneering forefathers of the profession may be coming to fruition a century later. The dual emphasis on sportive and supportive movement has returned to kinesiology. With this renewed emphasis on the study of forms of physical activity that relate not only to sportive "fun and games" but also to supportive activity for adequate daily functioning and the symbolic expressive features of human movement comes a change in the professional potential of the field.

## REFERENCES

Adelman, M. L. (1986). *A sporting time*. Champaign, IL: University of Illinois Press.

Betts, J. R. (September, 1953). The technological revolution and the rise of sport. *Mississippi Valley Historical Review, 15*, 231-256.

Feibleman, J.K. (1959). *Religious Platonism*. London: George Allen and Unwin Ltd.

Gulick, L. H. (1890). Physical education: A new profession. In *Proceedings of American Association for the Advancement of Physical Education, Cambridge and Boston, 1890*. Ithaca, NY: Andrus and Church.

Gutsmuths, J. C. F. (1800). *Gymnastics for youth*. London: J. Johnson.

Hartwell, E. M. (1886). *Physical training in American colleges and universities* (Circular of information of the Bureau of Education, No. 5-1885). Washington, DC: U. S. Government Printing Office.

Hartwell, E. M. (1899). The nature of physical training, and the best means of securing its ends. In I. Barrows(Ed.), *Physical training: A full report of the papers and discussions of the conference held in Boston in November 1899*. Boston: George H. Ellis.

Hetherington, C. W. (1925). Graduate work in physical education. *American Physical Education Review, 30*, 207-210, 262-268.

Howell, M. L., & Howell, R. (1988). Physical activities and sport in early societies. In E. Zeigler (Ed.), *History of physical education and sport* (pp. 1-56). Champaign, IL: Stipes Publishing.

Kroll, W. P. (1971). *Perspectives in physical education*. New York: Academic Press.

Metheny, E. (1965). *Connotations of movement in sport and dance*. Dubuque, IA: Wm. C. Brown Publishers.

Novak, M. (1976). *The joy of sports: End zones, bases, baskets, balls and the consecration of the American spirit*. New York: Basic Books.

Olivova, V. (1984). *Sports and games in the ancient world*. New York: St. Martin's Press.

Park, R. J. (1987). Sport history in the 1990s: Prospects and problems. In *American Academy of Physical Education Papers*, (Vol. 20, pp. 96-108). Champaign, IL: Human Kinetics.

Park R. J. (1989). The second 100 years: Or can physical education become the Renaissance field of the 21st century? *Quest, 41*, 1-27.

Rousseau, J. J. (1911). *Emile, on Education* (B. Forley, Trans.). London: J. M. Dent and Sons.

Sage, G. H. (1990). *Power and ideology in American sport: A critical perspective.* Champaign, IL: Human Kinetics.

Sargent, D. A. (1906). *Physical education.* Boston: Ginn.

Scanlon, T. F. (1984). Olympic dust, the Delphic laurel, and Isthmian toil: Horace and Greek athletics. *Arete: The Journal of Sport Literature, 1* (2), 163-178.

Scarborough, J. (1985). Galen on Roman amateur athletics. *Arete, 3,*(1), 171-176.

Smith, R. A. (1988). *Sports and freedom: The rise of big-time college athletics.* New York: Oxford University Press.

Sorokin, P. (1957). *Social and cultural dynamics.* Boston: Porter Sargent Publishers.

Spears, B., & Swanson, R. A. (1988). *History of sport and physical education in the United States.* Dubuque, IA: Wm. C. Brown Publishers.

Staley, S. C. (1937). The history of sport: A new course in the professional training curriculum. *Journal of Health and Physical Education, 8,* 522-525, 570-572.

Thompson, J. G. (1988). Political and athletic interaction in Athens during the sixth and fifth centuries B. C. *Research Quarterly for Exercise and Sport, 59*(3), 183-190.

Van Dalen, D. B., & Bennett, B. (1971). *A world history of physical education.* Englewood Cliffs, NJ:Prentice Hall.

Vertinsky, P. (1991). Science, social science, and the "hunger for wonders" in physical education: Moving toward a future healthy society. In *American Academy of Physical Education Papers, 24* (pp. 70-88). Champaign, IL: Human Kinetics.

Vuillier, G. (1898). *A history of dancing.* New York: D. Appleton and Co.

Winks, R. W. (1968). *The historian as detective.* New York: Harper and Row.

# SUGGESTED READING

Berryman, J., & Park, R. J. (Eds.). (1992). *Sport and Exercise Science: Essays in the History of Sports Medicine.* Urbana, IL: University of Illinois Press.

Gerber, E. W. (1971). *Innovators and Institutions in Physical Education.* Philadelphia: Lea and Febiger.

Gulick, L. H. (1904). *Physical Education By Muscular Exercise.* Philadelphia: P. Blakiston's Son and Co.

Haley, B. (1978). *The Healthy Body and Victorian Culture.* Cambridge, MA: Harvard University Press.

Howell, R. (Ed.). (1982). *Her Story in Sport.* Champaign, IL: Human Kinetics.

Kyle, D. G., & Stark, G. D. (Eds.). (1990). *Essays on Sport History and Sport Mythology.* College Station: Texas A. & M. Press.

Lucas, J. A. (1992). *Future of the Olympic Games.* Champaign, IL: Human Kinetics.

MacAloon, J. J. (1981). *This Great Symbol: Pierre de Coubestin and the Origins of the Modern Olympic Games.* Chicago: University of Chicago Press.

Malina, R. M., & Eckert, H. M. (Eds.). (1988). *Physical Activity in Early and Modern Populations.* Champaign, IL: Human Kinetics.

Mangan, J. A., & Park, R. J. (Eds.). (1987). *From "Fair Sex" to Feminism: Sport and the Socialization of Women in the Industrial and Post Industrial Eras.* London: Frank Cass.

Mangan, J. A., & Walvin, J. (Eds.). (1987), *Manliness and Morality: Middle-class Masculinity in Britain and America, 1800–1940.* New York: St. Martin's Press.

Oxendine, J. B. (1988). *American Indian Sports Heritage.* Champaign, IL: Human Kinetics.

Rader, B. G. (1990). *American Sports: From the Age of Folk Games to the Age of Televised Sports.* Englewood Cliffs, NJ: Prentice Hall.

Reiss, S. (1989). *City Games.* Urbana: University of Illinois Press.

Reiss, S. (Ed.). (1984). *The American Sporting Experience.* Champaign, IL: Human Kinetics.

Segrave, J. O. & Chu, D. (Eds.). (1988). *The Olympic Games in Transition.* Champaign, IL: Human Kinetics.

Spears, B. (1986). *Leading the Way: Amy Morris Homans and the Beginnings of Professional Education for Women.* New York: Greenwood Press.

Whorton, J. (1982). *Crusaders for Fitness: The History of American Health Reformers.* Princeton, NJ: Princeton University Press.

Zeigler, E. F. (1988). *History of Physical Education and Sport.* Champaign, IL: Stipes Publishing Co.

*An art and science that is applicable in the uncertainty of the real world.*

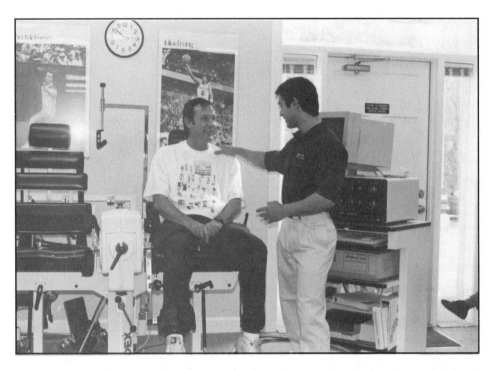

*"The human movement professions must go beyond the traditional specializations in teaching or in the use of sport to develop the nation's youth. . . . to serving all humans from womb to tomb. . . . to include the other therapeutic and habilitative processes of occupational and physical therapy. . . . and to capture ergonomics or human factors and form alignments with the health enhancement industry."*

(Ellis, 1989)

# The Future
# of Kinesiology

B y analyzing changes in the field throughout the course of history, carefully using demographic data, and selectively relying upon predictions of expert futurists, we can extrapolate trends toward the future of kinesiology. These trends suggest future directions within the academic study of human movement and career avenues that will open up for human movement professionals. The future of kinesiology in actuality will be many futures because of the diversity of departmental mission statements and the unique approaches of individual faculty members that typify modern higher education (Carnegie Council, 1976; Clark, 1983, 1987). Despite the disparities that currently exist and will continue to exist between programs, certain common denominators provide a basis for universally applicable predictions. These are: a shared culture, a mutual mission in higher education, and universal understanding of human movement.

The society that will unfold in the 21st century promises to yield great opportunity for the human movement professions. One of the purposes of this chapter is *to examine the intersections between society's future needs and professional opportunities for kinesiology*. The mission that kinesiology departments share is that of preparing high-quality professionals, individuals who have acquired certain basic understandings of human movement applicable in a variety of vocational and avocational settings. The responsibility that kinesiology departments recognize is to produce professionals who may move into occupations that are "based on a definable body of organized knowledge and expertise that derives from extensive academic training" and that involve a "moral commitment of service to the public" (Hatch, 1988).

Indicators of cultural change point toward a future society that places a premium upon health and well-being, that espouses personal fulfillment through physical activity, and that will amply reward the individuals who may serve the public by enhancing those qualities. The precise nature of these cultural changes and their expected impact upon kinesiology are discussed in this chapter.

The broad-based, integrated liberal arts paradigm and premises of knowledge, described in the first two parts of this book, will lead to a kinesiology graduate who is philosophically prepared to enter professional life, who understands the scientific, organismic functioning of the moving human body, and who appreciates the holistic, humanistic dimensions of humans moving. This kinesiology professional will have the versatility to be effective in a range of human movement-focused careers. The scope of opportunity that will beckon to kinesiology graduates in the future is examined using demographic data and trend analysis. Because of their significance to the kinesiology marketplace of the future, the trends discussed are illustrated in Figure 8.1. This illustration gives examples of how each of the developments in the different spheres of movement studied through kinesiology leads to potential employment markets. Kinesiologists may be employed in research, development, and implementation in each category.

## GENERAL TRENDS IN HIGHER EDUCATION

Two general trends currently evident in university kinesiology programs promise to radically affect the future path of the study of human movement. By changing the nature of the conceptualization of the discipline, they will open new horizons for kinesiology graduates in the job market.

## CURRICULUM CHANGES

Knowledge and skills in the curriculum will be reshaped to better reflect the understandings and needs of the real world. The argument for a more connected view of knowledge is not isolated within kinesiology; it has been a recurring theme throughout the undergraduate curriculum (Graff, 1991; Bok, 1986; Boyer, 1987). Activism in the relatively new and volatile field of kinesiology, however, has been particularly intense. The thrust toward narrower specializations in the 1960s and 1970s led to extensive debate in the 1980s (e.g. Greendorfer, 1987; Hoffman, 1985; Thomas, 1985), and finally to the action of the 1990s.

The most recent academic activism goes beyond name changes and adoption of a disciplinary liberal arts model to challenge the basic

THE PROMISE OF CONTEMPORARY KINESIOLOGY      PART III

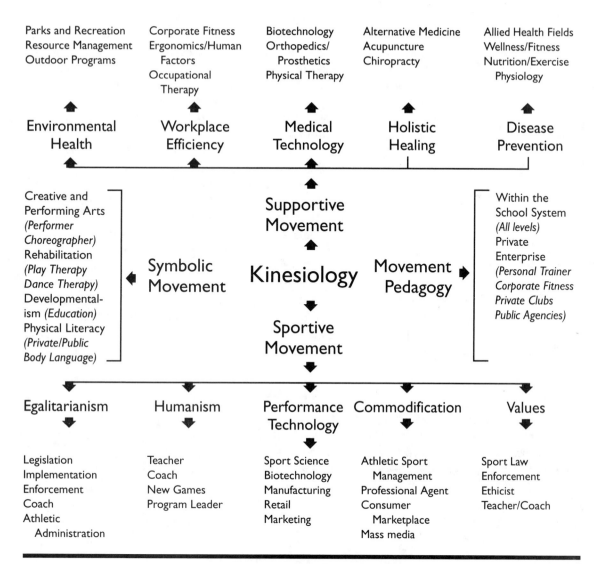

**FIGURE 8.1**

The Professional Promise of Kinesiology

structure of learning that had dominated the field since the 1960s. There is a unilateral call for a form of learning to transcend subject area barriers, form new academic alliances, and better represent the multi-faceted nature of knowing that exists beyond the confines of the university. Even within the higher education structure, recent evidence "strongly suggests broader preparation extending beyond the artificial boundaries of subdisciplinary study" (Zakrajsek & Pierce, 1993, p. 23).

The authors of that study concluded that "our research and doctoral granting institutions are not educating for a realistic college job market. . . . We have created a false market in our own self-image" (p. 23). A process of disconnected, overspecialized higher education that is deemed inappropriate for its own replication within the university certainly is not suitable for the general marketplace, in which multidimensional problems require multifaceted responses.

The American Academy of Kinesiology and Physical Education (1990) initiated the move away from the narrow subdisciplinary approach to the study of human movement, in its pronouncement that (in addition to changing their name to "kinesiology"), academic departments that study human movement in higher education should organize their curricula around 12 key concepts. Although these provide a starting point for a conceptual approach to kinesiology, without recognizing the levels of understanding with which they should be approached and the interrelated and complementary nature of the comprehension of these concepts, there is a danger of falling back into the traditional hierarchical approach. Adapting Gray Nabel's (1985) biological scheme, Roberta Park (1991) suggested five different levels of understanding, five different ways in which human movement should be studied:

*Level 5: Social aggregates — public policy, health, exercise, fitness, and sports; cultural, economic, and political factors influencing nutrition, exercise, and participation in sports; biomedical issues affecting health, exercise, and physical education in different epochs and cultures.*

*Level 4: The individual and small groups — aggressive and cooperative behaviors in sports settings; the psychosocial dynamics of the playground, psychological aspects of adherence to exercise, drugs, eating disorders, and aids to performance.*

*Level 3: Organ/System — the working heart; low hemoglobin, iron deficiency, and athletic performance; the oxygen transport system.*

*Level 2: Cellular — tissue and cell injuries; carbohydrates, oxidation, glucose and exercise; developmental biology and embryology.*

*Level 1: Subcellular — mitochondria, oxygen radicals, and exercise; nuclear protein degradation; calcium ion movements in cardiac tissue. (pp. 251-252)*

Whether this model, or one like it, is selected within a particular kinesiology department, the field is heading toward paradigms of learning that encompass the premises of a liberal arts approach. This entails "countering the fragmentation that keeps us from understanding the articulated whole" (Rintala, 1991, p. 275) by approaching human movement from a range of connected and overlapping perspectives.

From such a program of study will arise an art and science applicable in the uncertainty of the real world. The three premises of this prognosis are that kinesiology will produce a resilient and resourceful graduate, will emphasize experiential preparation within the context of the academic program, and will continue to be responsive to the changing needs of the culture. The successful application of acquired knowledge is essentially dependent upon the philosophic maturity of the kinesiology graduate. Only if individuals have been well schooled in philosophic skills (chapter 4) will they be able to apply their understanding of human movement (chapters 5 and 6) in an appropriate, logical, morally sound manner and to adapt to the changing conditions and challenges of their time.

## APPLICABILITY TO THE REAL WORLD

This transition away from the university to the professional setting may be eased by the familiarity bred by applied research. The political climate in higher education (which may be judged by funding and grant allocations) seems to increasingly support building bridges between academia and the professions. The future of applied research hinges upon the success of the academic discipline in developing and employing new paradigms of experimentation (Vertinsky, 1991, p. 84). When professionals accept experimentation as a valuable tool for improving practice and academics venture beyond the comfort of the highly controlled laboratory, kinesiology undergraduates are afforded a uniquely valuable way of learning by doing in the setting of their prospective careers.

The usefulness of academic preparation is closely allied with its breadth and its interconnectedness. The intellectual neutrality of the undergraduate program, which provides basic understanding of human movement without linking it explicitly to any one career field (to the detriment of all others) creates great professional potential. Michael Ellis (1990) recognized the scope of this potential in asserting:

*The human movement professions must go beyond the traditional specializations in teaching or in the use of sport to develop the nation's youth. The professions must be seen as serving all humans from womb to tomb. They should also not be limited to those professions using structured sport, dance, exercise, and play. The professions could easily expand over the next 25 years to include the other therapeutic and habilitative processes of occupational and physical therapy. The professions may also capture ergonomics or human factors and form alignments with the health enhancement industry. (p. 16)*

According to Ellis, then, movement professions that evolve from, and revolve around, supportive movement are a potential growth market for kinesiology.

## CHANGING EMPHASES IN SUPPORTIVE MOVEMENT

Cultural change, whether it be in the form of crises or more gradual evolution, is the catalyst that creates new consumer markets. Changing emphases in American society suggest trends that will continue to radically affect the consumer marketplace accessible to kinesiology. Demographic data indicate that the major growth area is in human movement professions that offer the kind of service to the general public that fosters greater efficiency and well-being in daily physical processes.

## PERSONAL HEALTH AND DISEASE PREVENTION

Patricia Vertinsky (1991) summarized the evidence that validates this trend:

*Changing demographic trends in North America show that a population that is becoming older, more heterogeneous, disproportionately female, and, by some current norms, healthy and vigorous, will demand a vast array of preventive health services both in the public sector and through private retailing. (pp. 70-71)*

Growing cultural recognition that pursuit of "the good life" is based upon the premise of good health spawned a wellness movement in American society that shows no signs of abating. Alexander McNeill (1987) attributed the growth of wellness programs to a network of economic, medical, and social influences. The confluence of these influences produced an approach to personal health, in its broadest sense, that stresses prevention rather than treatment of disease and puts the responsibility for health enhancement squarely on the consumer's shoulders. As McNeill observed:

*Wellness programs are built upon the premise that an individual should assume responsibility for his or her health and change lifestyle factors that contribute to chronic disease or other health risks. Wellness programs deal with physical, nutritional, psychological, intellectual, and metaphysical components of living. They involve a true integration of all components that constitute self. (p. 89)*

After completing a professional preparation program in kinesiology, with its emphasis upon the multidimensionality of human movement as an integral part of human being, graduates can enter the wellness field in a variety of career capacities (for example, in public or private agencies such as hospitals, schools, and welfare departments, in the corporate world of business, in health clubs and spas, or as self-employed consultants or personal trainers). Job descriptions range from generalized wellness program design, development, and leadership to more specific emphasis upon topics such as:

▶ medical screening and health risk appraisal.

▶ psychological well-being, including stress management, self-concept, and body-concept.

▶ social adjustment, such as coping with alienation and loneliness.

▶ behavioral adjustment (for example, alcohol and drug abuse).

▶ nutritional awareness, including diet and weight control.

▶ personal health, hygiene, and safety.

▶ environmental health, such as air pollution.

▶ occupational health analysis of workplace factors.

▶ spiritual health, highlighting personal metaphysical meanings and transcendent experience.

An allied field of employment is in research in private laboratories and agencies or in higher education that will lead to continuing development of the wellness field. Research may be focused in the exercise sciences (such as exercise biochemistry, exercise physiology, motor control, and biomechanics) or in the behavioral and sociocultural analysis of the human body and the meanings of movement.

Medical ideology is changing to open a window of opportunity for kinesiology graduates. Throughout the 20th century, reliance upon specialized forms of treatment, particularly surgery, and the prescription of drugs to combat disease had been the norm for the medical community. Reliable indicators suggest that a more holistic, naturalistic form of treatment is once again in vogue. Vertinsky (1991) observed that this approach is by no means new:

## HOLISTIC HEALING

*The idea that personal health could be improved by obeying natural laws (exercise, diet, sleep, sanguinity) has its roots in the classical Greek civilization, nourished in part by ancient convictions about the close connection between mind and body, but its blossoming in the first half of the 19th century attended that era's fascination with nature and personal freedom (Tesh, 1988, p. 21). (p.73)*

As evidence has surfaced concerning the psychosomatic nature of much disease and its treatment and the impact of lifestyle factors as cause and cure of many modern ailments, the pendulum has swung back toward treating the whole person. Consequently, kinesiology graduates, with their understanding of human anatomy, exercise science, and the behavioral aspects of physical activity, are increasingly gaining admission to medical schools and to post-graduate professional preparation leading to careers in fields such as physical therapy, occupational therapy, and cardiac rehabilitation, which emphasize movement as a modality.

In its search for effective treatment of the resilient diseases, such as AIDS and cancer, that plague western culture, the United States is supplementing traditional forms of medicine with various alternative healing modalities. The political establishment's willingness to countenance concepts, approaches, and methodologies previously considered too unconventional is evidenced by establishment within the structure of the National Institutes of Health of an office devoted to alternative medicine (by President Bill Clinton in 1993).

Many of these alternative approaches draw from previously untapped traditions from elsewhere in the world's medical community. Many Chinese practices, which have existed for more than 2,000 years, adopt a holistic approach to healing, emphasizing the synergistic energy forces of the body (chi) and the medicinal properties of natural organic substances. Another of humanity's most ancient approaches to healing, the Ayurvedic tradition of India, also is being tapped for insights that might be beneficial to western health. For example, in *Quantum Healing: Exploring the Frontiers of Mind/Body Medicine*, Chopra (1992) has combined western medicine and neuroscience with the insights of Ayurvedic theory, suggesting that the human body is controlled by a "network of intelligence" grounded in human reality, with the potential of defeating cancer, heart disease, and many of the problems associated with aging.

Eastern approaches such as these, and alternative healing methods emanating from advances in western science, are galvanizing change in western medicine. Learning to appreciate human movement and the mind-body relationship from a variety of disciplinary perspectives will prepare kinesiology graduates well for entry into emerging alternatives to traditional medicine, such as chiropracty, acupuncture, and other forms of holistic healing. Kinesiology graduates also will be qualified to seek out careers directed not upon healing the sick but, instead, upon enhancing the well-being of the healthy through alternative physical processes. Vertinsky (1991) predicted a continually growing number of clients for a service that brings about a sense of personal unity and enlightenment. She cited Mrozek (1987) and Solomon (1984) as examples of the increasing number of health seekers who seek exercise programs and holistic health practices, altered perceptions, cosmic affirmation, 'unity with nature,' and 'the integration of mind, body, and spirit for the attainment of whole health'" (p. 82).

Science and technology have assumed great importance in kinesiology and the health professions, as well as in every other facet of daily existence. Some critics (Park, 1991; McKay, Gore, & Kirk, 1990; Charles, 1979; Broekhoff, 1972) have suggested that "technocentric ideology" (Charles, 1979) has become too pervasive in current practice, leading to a "misplaced scientism" (Park, p. 249). This scientific approach is "misplaced" when the human dimensions of moving are subjugated by a mechanistic perspective that then dominates both the kinesiology curriculum and professional interactions with other people. A well balanced kinesiology program integrates humanistic appreciation of the mover with the scientific concepts and technological language that otherwise tend to produce a "reified" (Brockhoff, 1972) concept of human movement and the human body. This is illustrated in graphic detail in the following description:

*A self-balancing, 27 jointed adapter-base biped, an electrochemical reduction plant, integral with the segregated stowage of special energy extracts in storage batteries, for subsequent actuation of thousands of hydraulic and pneumatic pumps, with motors attached: 62,000 miles of capillaries, millions of warning signals, railroad and conveyor systems; crushers and cranes . . . and a universally distributed telephone system needing no service for 70 years if well managed; the whole extraordinary complex mechanism guided with exquisite precision from a turret in which are located telescopic and microscopic self-registering and recording range finders, a spectroscope, et cetera. (cited in McKay, Gore & Kirk, p. 60)*

Even though the language and ideology of technological scientism can be overly pervasive, the application of bioengineering concepts to the problems of human movement and, more broadly, to the nature of human being, is a fertile career field for kinesiologists in the future. Biomechanists find employment in any setting where structural realignment of bodily segments, or analysis of movement patterns, take place, such as in orthopedic surgery units and gait laboratories. Likewise, using engineering principles to overcome movement impediments through the design and manufacture of prosthetic devices, artificial limbs, and aids to enhance performance, such as hand-held outrigger skis for amputees is a marketable service. Computer applications, such as medical imaging, and software designs offer career opportunities for exercise scientists. The nature of the human body, growth processes, and movement potential is being altered by research and development in the field of biotechnology. This ongoing process is accessible through kinesiology, as graduates have a background in the science of the body, an understanding of the biochemical process of nutrition, knowledge of how science may alleviate disease, and an ethical concern for the future. Employed in what promises to be a monolithic enterprise to

## SCIENCE AND TECHNOLOGY IN HEALTH AND HEALING

restructure medicine, agriculture, and even the human body, kinesiology graduates are working in:

- ▶ the Human Genome Project (mapping chromosomes and designing treatments for disease on the basis of genetic blueprints).

- ▶ agricultural research (developing transgenic "mutant" livestock and crops, and experimenting with fertilizers and pesticides that are friendly to the environment but not to predators).

- ▶ genetic engineering (designing people through genetic manipulation and endocrinology).

## PHYSICAL EFFICIENCY IN THE WORKPLACE

In a fast-paced work world in which every minute counts, physical efficiency is an important consideration. Kinesiology professionals capitalize upon the personal and corporate goals of maximizing efficiency in two career contexts:

1. *Corporate fitness programs* are premised upon the notion that happy, healthy workers are efficient workers. Reducing absenteeism, enhancing employee health, increasing enthusiasm for the job and loyalty to the company — all carry underlying messages of efficiency and productivity to employers who hire kinesiology graduates to develop corporate fitness programs.

2. The study and enhancement of physical factors in the workplace fall under the purview of ergonomics. *Ergonomic analysis* is undertaken by kinesiology graduates with biomechanical understanding of physical efficiency, physiological comprehension of the capacities, needs, and limitations of the human body, and psychosocial awareness of motivational factors, behavioral considerations, and group dynamics.

## THE PHYSICAL ENVIRONMENT

The environmental radicalism of the 1960s matured through the decades to become a central issue in the mainstream of political life today. Opportunities for serving and preserving the environment today range from activist groups such as Greenpeace to centralized government bureaucracies such as the Environmental Protection Agency. Many students drawn to the study of the physical being also are interested, understandably, in the context of being physical: the physical environment. Students who have been active in leisure studies and outdoor recreation can enter professions that offer opportunities to experience nature firsthand in park and recreation agencies, marine resources, or outdoor adventure and outward bound programs. The growing public interest in ecological preservation, often linked to questions of environmental health, offers further scope for individuals with a background in human movement, health, and leisure studies. Employment opportunities range from agencies contructing ecological policies to groups with specific targeted agendas such as the Chesapeake Bay Foundation. An alternative is to work in the legal profession, interpreting and enforcing the environmental legal code.

A second form of environmentalism that has career ramifications for kinesiology graduates is concern for the qualities of an individual's environment that are necessary to produce personal health. One of the shortcomings of the wellness movement is that it targets a limited population of individuals whose personal environments allow them to exercise right, eat well, and profit from the services offered by wellness professionals. Alan Ingham (1985) broached this problem with sardonic humor:

*What do we have to offer the currently ill and about-to-be-ill segments of the population; those whose illnesses have more to do with workplace than lifestyle, with the ravages of unemployment rather than defects of character, with the cumulative effects of impoverishment — which is becoming increasingly feminized? Shall we say that they should aerobicize, jazzercise, and jog their problems away? Shall we counsel them to internalize the locus of control? (pp. 51, 54)*

Subsequently, Vertinsky (1991) noted:

*Pundits increasingly underline the downside of a health-promotion philosophy built upon personal responsibility for health, claiming that the lifestyle approach has ignored the more difficult but equally important problem of the social environment, which both creates some lifestyles and inhibits the maintenance of others (Crawford, 1980). (p. 80)*

In response to criticism of the shortcomings of a wellness philosophy that places individual responsibility for health upon the shoulders of those who are inevitably doomed to fail because of their personal environments, a new socioecological paradigm of health is emerging. Hal Lawson (1992) defined the key features of this new approach: "A socioecological conception of health calls attention to patterned interdependencies among individuals, groups, their lifestyle choices and stages, societal institutions, and the economic, spatial-communal, and natural-environmental contexts (i.e., human ecosystems)" (p. 111). Personal health is not only a personal responsibility but also a social issue. Kinesiology students, having studied humans moving from arts and science perspectives, are well prepared to enter this new field of health promotion, for, as Lawson suggested:

*Health promotion is the art and science of helping persons maintain or change their emotional, social, intellectual, spiritual, and physical characteristics: and, if necessary, changing social institutions and physical environments to bring them into greater harmony with ideals for healthy individuals and a healthy society. (p. 112)*

The opportunity for kinesiology graduates to enter this field will grow in the future. The nation's health care objectives for the year 2000 (Office of Disease Prevention and Health Promotion, 1991) placed a new emphasis upon health promotion and prevention and invited new initiatives and involvement from kinesiology and allied health fields. This broadened concept of health promotion is gaining in popularity in Canada too, as the Health and Welfare document *Achieving Health for All* (Epps, 1986) concluded:

*Health promotion implies a commitment to dealing with the challenges of reducing inequities, extending the scope of prevention, and helping people to cope with their circumstances. It means fostering public participation, strengthening community health services, and coordinating healthy public policy. Moreover, it means creating environments conducive to health in which people are better able to take care of themselves and to offer each other support in solving and managing collective health problems. (p. 12)*

The implication for professionals entering the field is that they will be in the business of empowering the socially disadvantaged through community-based programs, social service agencies, and public policy think-tanks. Kinesiology graduates could be prominent members in the future of this "huge, multifaceted profession in an age characterized by the need for cooperative efforts to confront global problems" (Vertinsky, 1991, p. 83).

## CHANGING EMPHASES IN SPORTIVE MOVEMENT

Sportive physical activity has gripped the nation and will continue to be a central focus of kinesiology and the source of employment for many students graduating with a degree in kinesiology. Career opportunities range from the primary participatory level of performing (including playing, coaching, and teaching) to the secondary level of sports consumerism (involving facilitating, managing, administering, spectating, litigating, researching, designing, selling and commentating). Career options built around these activities will continue to attract kinesiology graduates in the future, many of whom may have been attracted initially to the field by a love of sport fostered by their own athletic experiences and a desire to better understand the art and science of physical performance.

With their undergraduate background in the body of knowledge about human movement and their expertise derived from extensive academic training, kinesiology graduates enter the sports-related professions ready and able to serve the public. An alternative course is to opt for further graduate study to better prepare for fields such as sport management or sport law and research. Most trends in sportive activity have become well established during the growth period of the latter part of the 20th century, but recent, subtle changes in emphasis suggest new opportunities for professional involvement in the 21st century.

## EGALITARIANISM IN SPORT

The issue of whether all people, regardless of gender, race, age, handicapping condition, or talent should have the same access to, and treatment in, sport is being resolved more and more in the direction of egalitarianism. In recent decades, many athletes have become activists demanding equity. Women and minorities have campaigned for equal representation in the administrative hierarchy of the sports establishment. Legal precedents have been established that will lead to significant changes in high school sports, college athletics, and professional sport. Gender equity has been promoted by legal action — the passage of Title IX of the Education Amendments Act of 1972 and subsequent reaffirmation of its original intent and interpretation through the Civil Rights Restoration Act in 1988.

A logical conclusion to draw from this shift in emphasis is that some downscaling in the resources available to male sports will occur, but that massive growth will take place in programs, participation, and parity for females. Despite affirmative action effects, the burgeoning career field of female sports has not been, to this point, a windfall for women who aspire to coach and enter athletic administration. As George Sage (1990) noted:

*In high school, for example, in 1973-74 about 90% of high school girls sports were coached by women; in 1988-89 women coached less than 50% of the teams in the most popular girls sports . . . When Title IX was enacted in 1972, 90% to 100% of women's intercollegiate athletic teams were coached by females. . . . By 1988, less than half of the coaches of women's intercollegiate teams were women. (p. 51)*

As the thrust toward gender equity continues into the 21st century and as "the glass ceiling" limiting upward professional progress is shattered, career opportunities for women to perform, teach, coach, and organize athletic programs will increase significantly.

In contrast to the problem of gender equity, recent racial issues have hinged more upon the institutional racism that has limited access to leadership and management opportunities than upon the right to play. Certain elite sports still tend to limit the access of minorities, although even the most segregated of sports, golf, has relaxed its restrictions since the issue became front-page news when Hal Thompson, founder of the Shoal Creek Country Club, site of the 1990 PGA Championships, announced that accepting blacks into private clubs was "just not done in Birmingham, Alabama." In other sports, such as ice hockey and lacrosse, minorities are underrepresented because they did not have access to these sports in their youth. In the most popular American sports, however, minorities have achieved total integration as players.

The problem lies not so much in equal opportunity to perform (in which talent, not skin color, has become the primary determining criterion) as in equal and fair hiring practices within the hierarchy of sports management. Sage (1990) reported that "the stratification pattern for blacks has been similar to that for women with regard to sport leadership and management. Access for black athletes has expanded greatly in recent years, but very few blacks have been hired for positions high in the sports hierarchy" (p. 60). By 1989, the NFL had one black head coach and no black general managers. In 1990, only about 9% of the coaches and none of the general managers in major league baseball were black, and fewer than five NBA general managers were black. Black coaches have been equally scarce in intercollegiate athletics. "As of 1989, fewer than five major university football teams and 10 basketball teams were coached by blacks. Other sports have even fewer black coaches" (Sage, p. 60).

Challenges to the hegemonic system that historically has limited the opportunities of traditionally underprivileged groups continue to erode the status quo power bases and change the face of sport. Affirmative action programs and class action suits, the activism of groups representing the interests of women and minorities (such as the Rainbow Commission for Fairness in Athletics), and the increasing unwillingness of underprivileged individuals in sport to accept roles that are "second best" are indications that sport is becoming more egalitarian.

Other populations of individuals who typically have been neglected in the past are also gaining access to sports participation. Since the passage of the Education for All Handicapped Children Act of 1975 (Public Law 94-142) and the reaffirmation and expansion of its principles in 1990 through the Individuals with Disabilities Education

Act (Public Law 101-476), schools, colleges, and public sport and recreation agencies have begun to expand their programs to include special populations with disabilities either in the mainstream of activities or in alternative programs, such as Special Olympics.

Sport, which used to be considered the province of the young, is diversifying to become popular with the young-at-heart. More people of all ages are participating in recreational activities and organized sports programs. People once considered too elderly to be vigorously active are enjoying the most strenuous and adventurous of physical pursuits sponsored by recreation departments, elderhostels, and the Golden Olympics organization, among others. As Joseph Levy (1983) noted, "With one in every six citizens over 65 years of age by the year 2001 (as is predicted), planning for this group will be mandatory" (p. 14). If the gradual transformation of sport envisioned by Sage continues into the 21st century, it will present kinesiology graduates with an array of new employment possibilities. The egalitarian nature of the sport system of the future may include:

*The values of a decent, progressive sport system (which) will center on equality. . . . This egalitarian sport system will provide adequate facilities and equipment for everyone, regardless of means . . . In a society committed to egalitarianism, active participation is encouraged and adequate resources are universally available. . . . Arbitrary distinctions of sex, race, and age will cease to function as forms of oppression or criteria for limiting sport opportunities. (Sage, 1990, pp. 216-217).*

The increasing egalitarianism of the sport system will lead to a higher level of humanism in sport. Equality of rights and opportunities for every member of society regardless of capacity, race, creed, age, or gender will inspire self-determination. The capacity and empowerment of self-determination are a basic premise of a humanistic vision of sport in the future. As Joseph Levy (1983) articulated this idea:

## A HUMANISTIC APPROACH TO SPORT AND LEISURE

*I see on the horizon the emergence of a new sport and leisure ethic based on humanistic principles and values. It will speak to the individual as a member of society — throughout life. Sport and leisure in tandem with community and personal values must contribute toward the achievement of an optimal quality of life. (p. 14)*

This trend toward humanism found its earliest expression in the New Games movement initiated during the social ferment of the 1960s. Steward Brand and other counter-culture figures established the New Games Foundation in the San Francisco area to change the way people played by replacing competitive sports with cooperative, no-win/no-lose forms of play. The foundation continues to be instrumental in creating an atmosphere of fun and relaxed voluntary participation through weekend workshops throughout the country for recreation specialists, educators, and health-care professionals.

During this same period, concern for self-development leading to higher awareness, was the theme of the Esalen Institute in California and at other locations.

Emphasis upon "the inner game" and enlightenment through various exercise forms naturally led to preoccupation with various forms of eastern activity. Eastern martial arts have continued to grow in popularity in the United States since that time, though some, particularly judo and karate, have been largely divested of their essential philosophical nature. Acknowledging the shortcomings of the traditional competitive sports model, many members of the counter-culture in the 1960s either "turned off" or "dropped out." In many cases, these who were turned off by their failures in competitive participation became spectators. As Levy (1983) observed:

*Mounting psychological evidence indicates that North American adults adopt the passive sports spectator role earlier than their European counterparts because their childhood sport "failure" experiences condition them to avoid direct sports involvement. (p. 13)*

Through the decades since the turbulent 1960s, many people have dropped out of competitive team sports and have found in their place an alternative form of physical fulfillment through individual lifetime sports. Activities that may be enjoyed through the lifespan continue to be a growing marketplace for kinesiology graduates. In particular, outdoor adventure activities such as wind surfing, rock climbing, rafting, canoeing, and kayaking are enjoying a growth spurt that shows no sign of abating.

In contrast to the humanism of the 1960s, which centered on self-actualization and led to the narcissism of the "me generation" of the 1970s, the humanism of the future involves an element of commitment to the environment. Many activities becoming popular today, such as rock climbing, require a high level of cooperation and trust in the immediate environment (which includes belayers and spotters as well as ropes and the rock face). These *eco-sports* also create humanistic interdependence, an understanding that "people, plants, and animals should be treated as interdependent components in the ecology of life" (Levy, 1983, p. 14). The growth of activities that rely upon nature and the influence of nontraditional activities derived from eastern and native American Indian heritages, which revere nature in various ways, promotes a lifestyle in harmony with nature rather than one based upon mastery and manipulation of the environment. This growing emphasis upon humanism in sport and leisure activities will provide kinesiology professionals in the 21st century with an array of opportunities to develop and lead cooperative games, eastern martial arts, lifetime activities, adventure education, and eco-sports.

Although eco-sports, with their emphasis on natural movement and harmony with the environment, are becoming more popular, most modern sports use artificial means and synthetic equipment to enhance performance. The impact of technology ranges from advances in safety (such as the football helmet) and comfort (such as the running shoe) to dramatic evolution in equipment (such as the Fiberglass pole) and inventions that have made a sport possible (such as the universal mast foot of a sailboard, which allows the rig to rest on the water while the board stays upright).

## THE TECHNOLOGY OF PERFORMANCE

Ever since the 19th century, when much American progress hinged upon ingenuity and inventiveness, the American public has been enamored with technology. Sport provides a natural venue for technological experimentation. The results can be spectacular, and the rewards significant. Many kinesiology graduates are employed in the areas of equipment design and performance enhancement now, and, as Cavanaugh (1987) suggested, "It is reasonable to expect that the dividends will be larger in the future as more and more areas of application are realized" (p. 118). Biomechanists have contributed significantly to the sophistication of the sport shoe (Frederick, 1984; Nigg & Kerr, 1983), the aerodynamic qualities of equipment, and clothing design in cycling (Kyle, 1986) and to the development of software packages that analyze and improve the movement patterns of athletes.

The technology of performance enhancement extends beyond biomechanical parameters to the intersection of physiology and psychology. For example, advanced computerized techniques such as holograms (three-dimensional laser images), can be combined with electrical data on muscle functioning to provide invaluable feedback that can be used in tandem with sports psychology, to extend current limits of human performance. As Harris (1987) noted:

*The research in exercise and sport psychology is on the threshold of making a significant and meaningful contribution to greater insight and understanding of an integrated involvement in exercise and sport. The extension of human abilities will be reached only when we find ways of integrating and amplifying the increasing new technologies and techniques now being developed. (p. 45)*

Because the limits of human performance are highly correlated with the frontiers of the mind, sport psychology has become an ever more popular choice of profession for graduating kinesiologists. Sport psychologists are being employed wherever sport is important. Their numbers are growing in the public school system, in colleges, in the professional sport establishment, and in training centers for elite athletes such as the Olympic training center at Colorado Springs, Colorado. Their job descriptions run the gamut of researching, counseling, and organizing players and sport systems. They address topics such as motivation and attitudes, biofeedback, psychological aspects of injury, anxiety and performance, arousal and performance, cognitive, situational, and social factors in sport, imagery, attention styles, personality factors, mental preparation, body imagery, aggression, and organizational and interpersonal dynamics.

The growth in high-tech sport in improving performance standards are causing a ripple effect throughout society. The trend toward egalitarianism is ensuring that technology will continue to reach into the hinterlands of American society, touching the lives of special populations including children, elderly people, and those with certain motor impairments. In the process, it will create employment opportunities for those with a kinesiology background and a commitment to serve these groups of people.

## THE COMMODIFICATION OF SPORT

The trend toward commodification of sport, in which services and goods are produced for commercial gain, dates back to the emergence of modern capitalism. The recent expansion of amateur and professional spectator sports and the boom in participatory sports have given impetus to this trend throughout the sports industry. At the professional level, capital investors own and organize their sport businesses with the aim of accumulating capital. At another level, nonprofit organizations such as schools and universities adopt a similar model of commodification but with the intent of only breaking even. Athletic administration within nonprofit agencies requires the same managerial acumen and attention to the bottom line as the professional sports industry.

The secondary marketplace of associated goods and services provides an opportunity for businesses to accumulate capital through indirect participation in sports. An individual with the qualifications of an undergraduate degree in kinesiology and appropriate further training is well prepared to enter secondary markets such as the sporting goods industry (research and development, manufacture, and retail), the mass media (sport on television, in newspapers and magazines), the advertising industry (designing or buying sports advertising, sponsoring events), and other sports-related concerns (promoters, the travel business, hotels and restaurants at host sites).

A promising and popular route to employment in this general area is through graduate programs in sport and fitness management. One measure of the viability of this course of action is the U. S. Bureau of Labor Statistics ("Jobs," 1985), which indicated that, from 1985 to 1995, only computer electronics (35%), health care (29%), and high tech (28%) industries would exceed the projected employment growth of leisure and recreation services, which includes sport management. True to form, the demand for suitably qualified management has continued to increase throughout the range of sport settings, in which sport is treated as an activity, a modality, a service, a tenant, or a sales product (Vander Smissen, 1987). Kinesiology graduates are employed "in the schools, in public recreation, in YWCAs and YMCAs, in the military, in amateur sports, in retirement villages and senior centers, in resorts, and hotels, in employee recreation, in business and industry" (p. 102).

Leadership skills also are necessary to administer sport, or exercise, as a modality (a treatment for various physiological, behavioral, and emotional problems such as high stress levels, the need for cardiac rehabilitation, obesity, and many lifestyle diseases). Qualitatively different managerial skills are necessary to manage sport as a service enterprise in settings such as racquet clubs, golf country clubs, marinas, fitness centers, swimming pools, and health clubs. The skills of management include balancing the budget while offering an acceptable level of service, and marketing and promoting these services while keeping abreast of changes in the industry. One form of management requires the skills of a landlord when sport is the tenant of a large stadium, arena, or sport complex.

In other contexts, sport is a sales product (to the extent that its equipment, apparel, and skills are bought and sold in the marketplace by those with appropriate entrepreneurial training.) The retail market, however, extends far beyond selling. In addition to salespersons, a wide career field is opening up for technical writers and instructional media experts. "Closely related is the advertising field with its generous use of sport as an advertising medium" (Van der Smissen, 1987, p. 105). As the trend toward commodification of sport escalates into the future, the demand for kinesiology students trained in sport management will continue to grow.

Some trends have emerged in recent years suggesting that ethical practice in sport will continue to receive more attention. Foremost is

**VALUES IN SPORT**

the growing public concern about standards and actions culture-wide. In the wake of well publicized abuses in politics, business, medicine, and research, the general public naturally is skeptical. Consequently, calls for government commissions to investigate illegal or unethical practices, scandals broken by investigative reporting of the media, and challenges within professional associations to establish and abide by their own codes of ethics, are all becoming more common. This nation-wide sensitivity to questions of values has compounded the problems of sport. In recent years sport has been plagued by a rash of abuses that seem to threaten its very integrity. The incisiveness of the media in exposing ethical lapses in sport has brought to the public eye a series of scandals and allegations concerning highly visible figures from the world of sports.

Many contemporary critics suggest that the future health of sport is connected intimately with the ability of the sports establishment to curb abuses and impose ethical standards on participants. Of the many issues that have arisen to threaten the integrity of sport in the 21st century, 10 of the most pressing are:

1. Overemphasis on winning (win at all costs).

2. Underemphasis on equality (access, opportunity, treatment).

3. The role of technology (reflected in commonly asked questions such as: Should performance-enhancing aids be legal if they are available only to a privileged minority? What limits should be placed on "psychodoping" technology, used to experiment with the mind and break down psychological barriers? Might biotechnology be used in sport to manufacture superior athleticism through genetic manipulation?).

4. Violence as a strategy for victory.

5. The erosion of sportsmanship.

6. Permissible limits of spectator fanaticism.

7. Manipulation, exploitation, and alienation of some athletes.

8. The competition between chemists (in developing and administering ergogenic aids).

9. The role of sport in education.

10. Questions of personal morality (e.g., gambling, abuse of celebrity status in personal relationships, drug use and alcohol abuse, licentiousness, and profanity).

Kinesiology graduates who are interested in these ethical questions can find their niche in the sport marketplace in various settings including agencies established to oversee sport, or the sport establishment itself, higher education, or regulatory agencies such as the National Collegiate Athletic Association.

The final arbiter of moral issues is the legal system. Sport law is becoming a recognized subfield within the legal profession because of the growing demand for specialists in social issues, such as gender equity, suits stemming from sport-related injury as a result of negligence, professional contracts and disputes, and sport violence. Regardless of their vocational choice, kinesiology graduates, with their philosophical background, will be in a position to lead a resurgence in values in sport, through their exemplary avocational, recreational participation.

## CHANGING EMPHASES IN SYMBOLIC MOVEMENT

Just as interest in sportive and supportive aspects of human movement is spreading through society, creating professional opportunities in its wake, symbolic movement also is undergoing a renaissance. As Moore and Yamamoto (1988) observed, "In addition to the burgeoning interest in the functional aspects of body movement, there is a renewed concern for its expressive properties" (p. 295).

## THE CREATIVE AND PERFORMING ARTS

One indicator of the growing national interest in expressive movement is the proliferation of professional companies of performers of various forms of dance and other movement arts. And the popularity of physical activities near the intersection of sportive and symbolic forms of movement, such as synchronized swimming and rhythmic gymnastics, attests to the public fascination with expression in and through movement. The resurgence of interest in dance has professional implications for those in kinesiology who aspire to be performers, choreographers, and event facilitators. It also has avocational applications throughout the culture, as Franziska Boas (1971) commented:

*At last, dance in modern society is acquiring the natural function which it had and still has in these less mechanized and less guilt-ridden cultures. . . . Men and women, both young and old, have discovered that participation in dance activity is not limited to the professional dancer but that they may find a renewal of life, a stimulus to creative action and certainly a better understanding of the intricacies of human nature through actual doing. (pp. i, ii)*

## THE REHABILITATIVE QUALITIES OF PHYSICAL EXPRESSION

During the past 30 years, symbolic movement in rehabilitation is most apparent in the fields of dance therapy and, to a lesser extent, play therapy. Through structured movement experiences, individuals with emotional and psychological disturbance are given therapy based on the regenerative power of self-expression through movement. Although the roots of this healing process date back to primal cultures, harnessing the transformative power of movement is a recent innovation in western psychotherapy. Treatment traditionally has centered on words, and occasionally chemicals, but as the trend towards alternative holistic healing processes continues to make inroads into western medicine, recognition of the importance of treating the whole person will continue to grow. Students with undergraduate preparation in the functioning of the human body and its interrelationships with the mind, and appropriate further training in psychotherapeutic methodologies, are ideally suited for professions that offer therapy through movement.

## THE DEVELOPMENTAL QUALITIES OF SYMBOLIC HUMAN MOVEMENT

The developmental use of symbolic movement is having its most obvious impact in education. Dance in the curriculum is not new. As Rudolph Laban (1974) suggested, "Formerly such dances were one of the main means of schooling the young to adapt themselves to the habits and customs of their forebears" (p. 54). Yet, for many years dance and other forms of expressive movement fell from favor in education as formalized physical training and athletics held sway.

Recently, more expressive forms of educational gymnastics and more creative modes of movement education have gained popularity in the gymnasium. Dance is even finding its way into the training regimen of many athletic teams (some NFL teams incorporate ballet into their game preparation). Educational philosophy is turning toward an approach that fosters the total, integrated concept of development, because of changing perceptions of the purposes of schooling. As Best (1982) summarized it: "If children do not acquire certain techniques, whether of language, the arts, or any other subjects, they are deprived of certain possibilities for freedom of expression and individuality" (p. 285). Numbered among these techniques are the skills of self-expression through movement (Stinson, 1985). Consequently, dance is being taught as an art form in schools and academies with increasing frequency, with the aim of developing techniques or properties including rhythm, symmetry, harmony, balance, continuity, unity, and contrast (Arnold, 1988, p. 100).

## PHYSICAL LITERACY

The skills of self-expression through bodily actions are as necessary to the general population as they are to special populations who need therapy or depend upon sign language to communicate. The ability to communicate clearly through body language has profound effects upon interpersonal relationships. Defining and refining movement patterns to enhance communication capacity is a field of enterprise relatively untapped by kinesiology. Yet, techniques that might enhance personal charisma, interpersonal appeal, and the powers of persuasion promise to be highly marketable in the 21st century. With a thorough understanding of human movement, professionals in "the body business" are singularly well placed to capitalize upon the potential growth market in how to communicate effectively through body language.

Nonverbal communication has significant professional applications beyond this "self-help" market, in which physical literacy is promoted as a form of personl enchancement. Service industries, ranging from medicine to education and from insurance to banking, are predicated upon trust and cooperation between producer and consumer. This relationship will continue to be developed primarily through one-on-one contact in meetings and consultations, even in the future society of faxes and fiberoptics. (For example, recognition of the importance of visual contact in communication has prompted the telecommunications industry to develop plans to replace the impersonal nature of the telephone with interactive video technology to allow visual images and body language.) The quality of this relationship hinges in large part upon the clarity of physical messages that accompany words during meetings. Dale Leathers (1986, pp. 7-10), suggested that body language is a crucial feature of communciation for the following reasons:

1. Nonverbal factors are the major determinants of meaning in the interpersonal context.

2. Feelings and emotions are revealed more accurately by nonverbal than by verbal means.

3. The nonverbal portion of communication conveys meanings and intentions that are relatively free of deception and distortion.

4. Nonverbal cues serve a metacommunicative function that is indispensable in attaining high-quality communication.

5. Nonverbal cues represent a much more efficient means of communication than verbal cues.

6. Nonverbal cues represent the most suitable vehicle for suggestions.

Figuring out the movement vocabulary that constitutes body language and then translating that knowledge into a marketable product, an educational program, and even a software package is one of the challenges of the future for those in the human movement field.

## CHANGING EMPHASES IN MOVEMENT PEDAGOGY

Teaching others to move efficiently and effectively is the time-honored profession that the preponderance of physical education students traditionally gravitated toward and it still attracts a large proportion of kinesiology graduates. In the latter part of the 20th century, physical education in the school system has not veered from its emphasis upon play, games, and sports, prompting critics such as Ravitch (1983) to suggest that:

*Schools in the year 2000 will bear the same relationship to the schools of 20 years ago. If we consider how little schools have changed since 1966, it seems utopian to predict that all schools in the foreseeable future might be as good as the very best schools of today. (p. 320)*

Change is not necessarily desirable, particularly when a system is functioning efficiently, but, in the case of the school system, demographic evidence suggests that physical education is being deemphasized and even eliminated in many areas. In addition, the "traditional and primarily custodial culture of physical education" is being "reinforced by successive generations of physical educators" (Templin, 1987, p. 59) and more physical educators are leaving their jobs in the first three years than are continuing. From a process of data extrapolation, Locke (1986) concluded:

*We can reasonably expect to find that of every 10 students entering professional preparation, fewer than three will remain in physical education three years after graduation. If they are like other teachers, of those who remain, most will be making plans to depart. (p. 90)*

Despite these gloomy predictions, there are signs that the enterprise of education is healthy.

## EXPANSION WITHIN THE SCHOOL SYSTEM

Although acquiring athletic skills and executing them in competitive contests remains the central aim of many programs, other priorities are emerging on the school scene. Curricular initiatives are making incursions into both the supportive and the symbolic domains of movement.

In the supportive domain, health-related fitness is assuming more importance in programs that emphasize wellness skills, lifestyle concepts, and lifetime activities. One indicator of the growing desire of school physical educators to be involved in the health-related fitness movement is the fervor with which the American Alliance of Health, Physical Education, Recreation and Dance lobbied Congress in 1993 to be included in the national initiative *Healthy People 2000*. Symbolic movement is gaining attention through the inclusion of dance in some curricula and in the standards-setting process of the national education plan established in the early 1990s.

In addition, many elementary schools are adopting the movement education philosophy developed in progressive schools in England. Its thematic emphasis upon problem solving and movement exploration encourages students to discover their own physical potential in a non-threatening atmosphere where standards are relative and competition is deemphasized.

A second area of expansion is in the quality of teaching and teacher education. Although "teachers in the field continue to teach much as they always have, quite untouched by research findings . . . there seems to be good cause for some guarded optimism about the long-term impact of new knowledge on teaching and teacher education" (Locke, 1987, p. 85). Among the innovations that will enhance the quality of instruction are research-based teaching texts, training modules for teacher effectiveness, and qualitative ethnographic research methodologies that more clearly assess the nature of the learning taking place in physical education.

From qualitative field studies, research into the "hidden curriculum," and task analyses come unambiguous evidence that "the functional curriculum for many students is substantially different from the formal intentions of the teacher" (Locke, 1987, p. 87). Armed with the knowledge that "many students in the gym are neither doing the tasks we assign nor learning the things we intend" (p. 87), new teachers and coaches are seeking to effect change, to more closely align principle with practice, and ultimately to improve the quality and scope of learning in physical education, kindergarten through 12th grade.

## MOVEMENT EDUCATION OUTSIDE THE SCHOOL SYSTEM

Education by no means is confined to the school environs or to people of school age. Although the demand for physical education teachers and coaches for the school system, will continue, the growth market of the 21st century is beyond the school walls. Kinesiology graduates are teaching in the health care field, the leisure industry, and the military. Employment in the private sector requires a mindset and a level of understanding of human movement that will appeal to sophisticated consumers of all ages. Whereas a school class is a captive audience usually satisfied with "team games and sports requiring neoadolescent vigor and foolhardiness," the business of movement education requires "people oriented to the enhancement of individuals throughout the lifespan, rather than people attracted by the glamour of elitism" (Ellis, 1987, p. 80). Fostering athletic excellence is only one of the vocational avenues open to practitioners beyond the school walls, through involvement in youth sports programs or skill enhancement through clinics, clubs, or private lessons. Movement educators in the private sector also use physical activity as a modality, as a health benefit, and as a means to find fulfillment.

Certain characteristics of this growing marketplace dictate the criteria for success. Because the information revolution of the past decades has led to a level of consumer demystification (Naisbitt, 1982), clients are becoming more sophisticated. They have access through information technology such as personal computers to the information that was the privileged purview of professionals in prior years. They often understand wellness principles, nutritional knowledge, the fundamentals of skill production, and the constituents of good health. They may be older, more demanding, and more idiosyncratic, requiring individualized attention, consultation, and in-depth knowledge of human movements. Kinesiology graduates are employed in a range of careers that depend upon pedagogical expertise. For example, one might be a personal trainer (involved in exercise prescription and compliance), and another could be a corporative fitness executive (concerned with program development and management). The progressive segmentation of the market to provide greater client choice has opened a window of opportunity for well informed kinesiology graduates. Ambitious and aggressive entrepreneurs can discover a market niche providing unique services to clientele of all ages. Alternatively, already proven programs can be provided through franchising, which Ellis (1987) described as "a recently developed strategy for exploiting the opportunities created by market segmentation, and . . . for helping people start up and operate small businesses that serve a local need" (p. 80). Information acquisition through research, and information dissemination through teaching, will continue to offer kinesiologists vocational opportunities in and beyond the formal structure of education.

**SUMMARY**

Trends to the future suggest that a good undergraduate program in kinesiology will provide excellent preparation for living and working in the 21st century. The liberal arts approach to the study of human movement, which emphasizes skills and knowledge that are enlightening in any setting, transcends the perimeters of academic departments and the parameters of specific jobs. It imparts to kinesiology students an intellectual understanding of the body and its functioning and of the human dimensions of moving and being that are necessary to enter an array of professions.

With appropriate graduate and professional study and on-the-job internship experience, kinesiology students will find that their services are in demand. For as long as preventive medicine, proactive health, and personal well-being; sport, recreation, and leisure; physical creativity, self-expression, and dance; and teaching, learning, and understanding movement processes remain important in the culture, kinesiology will provide invaluable undergraduate preparation for a rewarding personal and professional lifetime.

# REFERENCES

American Academy of Kinesiology and Physical Education. (1990). Resolution on Kinesiology. In *Academy Papers* (Vol. 23, p. 104). Champaign, IL: Human Kinetics.

Arnold, P. J. (1988). *Education, movement and the curriculum.* New York: Falmer Press.

Best, D. (1982). Can creativity be taught? *British Journal of Educational Studies, 30*(2), 280-294.

Boas, F. (1972). *The function of dance in human society.* New York: Dance Horizons.

Bok, D. (1986). *Higher learning.* Cambridge, MA: Harvard University Press.

Boyer, E. L. (1987). *The undergraduate experience in America: The Carnegie Foundation for the Advancement of Teaching.* New York: Harper and Row.

Broekhoff, J. (1972). Physical education and the reification of the human body. *Gymnasium, 9*, 4-11.

Carnegie Council on Education. (1976). *A classification of institutions of higher education.* Berkeley, CA: University of California Press.

Cavanagh, P. R. (1987). The cutting edge in biomechanics. In *American Academy of Physical Education Papers* (Vol. 20, pp. 115-119). Champaign, IL: Human Kinetics.

Charles, J. M. (1979). Technocentric ideology in physical education. *Quest, 31*(2), 277-284.

Chopra, D. (1992). *Quantum healing: Exploring the frontiers of mind/body medicine.* New York: Bantam New Age Books.

Clark, B. R. (1983). *The higher education system: Academic organization in cross-national perspective.* Berkeley, CA: University of California Press.

Clark, B. R. (Ed.). (1987) *The academic profession: National, disciplinary, and institutional settings.* Berkeley, CA: University of California Press.

Crawford, R. (1980). Healthism and the medicalization of everyday life. *International Journal of Health Sciences,* 10(13), 365-388.

Ellis, M. J. (1987). The business of physical education. In J. D. Massengale, (Ed.), *Trends toward the future in physical education,* (pp. 69-86). Champaign, IL: Human Kinetics.

Ellis, M. J. (1990). Reactions to "The Body of Knowledge: A Common Core." In *American Academy of Physical Education Papers* (Vol. 23, pp. 13-16), Champaign, IL: Human Kinetics.

Epps, J. (1986). *Achieving health for all: A framework for health promotion.* Ottawa, Canada: Health and Welfare Canada.

Frederick, E. C. (1984). *Sport shoes and playing surfaces: Biomechanical properties.* Champaign, IL: Human Kinetics.

Graff, G. (1991). Colleges are depriving students of a connected view of scholarship. *Chronicle of Higher Education,* 37(22), A48.

Harris, D. V. (1987). Frontiers in psychology of exercise and sport. *In American Academy of Physical Education Papers* (Vol. 20, pp. 26-41). Champaign, IL: Human Kinetics.

Hatch, N. O. (1988). Introduction: The professions in a democratic culture. In N. O. Hatch (Ed.), *The professions in American history* (pp. 1-13). Notre Dame, IN: University of Notre Dame Press.

Ingham, A. (1985). From public issue to personal trouble: Well-being and the fiscal crisis of the state. *Sociology of Sport Journal, 2*(1), 43-55.

"Jobs of the Future." (1985). *U. S. News and World Report,* December 23, pp. 40-45.

Kyle, G. (1986). Equipment design criteria for the competitive cyclist. In E. R. Burke (Ed.), *Science of cycling* (pp. 137-144). Champaign, IL: Human Kinetics.

Laban, R. (1974). *The language of movement.* Boston: Plays Inc.

Lawson, H. A. (1992). Toward a socioecological conception of health. *Quest, 44*, 105-121.

Leathers, D. G. (1986). *Successful nonverbal communication: Principles and applications.* New York: Macmillan.

Levy, J. (1983, April). Toward a humanistic approach to sports and leisure: Implications beyond 2001. *Journal of Physical Education, Recreation and Dance*, pp. 12-14.

Locke, L. F. (1987). The future of research on pedagogy: Balancing on the cutting edge. In *American Academy of Physical Education Papers* (Vol. 20, pp. 83-95). Champaign, IL: Human Kinetics.

McKay, J., Gore, J. M., & Kirk, D. (1990). Beyond the limits of technocratic physical education. *Quest, 42*(1), 52-76.

McNeill, A. (1987). Wellness programs and their influence on professional preparation. In J. D. Massengale (Ed.), *Trends toward the future in physical education* (pp. 85-94). Champaign, IL: Human Kinetics.

Moore, C., & Yamamoto, K. (1988). *Beyond words: Movement observation and analysis*. Philadelphia: Gordon and Breach.

Mrozek, D. J. (1987). The scientific quest for physical culture and the persistent appeal of quackery. *Journal of Sport History, 14*(1), 76-86.

Nabel, G. J. (1985). Order and human biology. *American Journal of Medicine, 78*, 545-548.

Naisbitt, J. (1982). *Megatrends: Ten new directions transforming our lives*. New York: Warner Books.

Nigg, B. M., & Kerr, B. A. (Eds.) (1983). *Biomechanical aspects of sport shoes and playing surfaces*. Calgary, Alberta, Canada: University of Calgary Press.

Office of Disease Prevention and Health Promotion. (1991). *Health care objectives for the year 2000*. Washington, D.C.

Park, R. J. (1991). On tilting at windmills while facing Armageddon. *Quest, 43*(3), 247-259.

Ravitch, D. (1983). On thinking about the future. *Phi Delta Kappan, 64*, pp. 317-320.

Rintala, J. (1991, December). The mind-body revisited. *Quest, 43*(3), 260-279.

Sage, G. H. (1990). *Power and ideology in American sport: A critical perspective*. Champaign, IL: Human Kinetics.

Solomon, H. A. (1984). *The exercise myth*. New York: Harcourt Brace Jovanovich.

Stinson, S. W. (1985). Curriculum and the morality of aesthetics. *Journal of Curriculum Theorizing, 6*(3), 66-83.

Templin, T. J. (1987). Some considerations for teaching physical education in the future. In J. D. Massengale (Ed.), *Trends toward the future in physical education* (pp. 51-68). Champaign, IL: Human Kinetics.

Tesh, S. N. (1988). *Hidden arguments: Political ideology and disease prevention policy*. New Brunswick NJ: Rutgers University Press.

Van der Smissen, B. (1987). Sport management: Its potential and some developmental concerns. In J. D. Massengale (Ed.), *Trends toward the future in physical education* (pp. 95-120). Champaign, IL: Human Kinetics.

Vertinsky, P. (1991). Science, social science and the "hunger for wonders" in physical education: Moving toward a future healthy society. In *American Academy of Physical Education Papers* (Vol. 24, pp. 70-88). Champaign, IL: Human Kinetics.

Zakrajsek, D., & Pierce, W. (1993, May-June). Academic preparation and the academic consumer. *Journal of Physical Education, Recreation and Dance, 64*(5), 20-23, 31.

## SUGGESTED READING

Association for Fitness in Business, (1992). *Guidelines for Employee Health Promotion Programs*. Champaign, IL: Human Kinetics.

Austin, N. & Peters, T. (1985). *A Passion for Excellence*. New York: Random House.

Barette, G. T., Feingold, R. S., Rees, C. R., & Pieron, M. (Eds.). (1987). *Myths, Models, and Methods in Sport Pedagogy*. Champaign, IL: Human Kinetics.

Benne, K. D. (1990). *The Task of Post-contemporary Education: Essays in Behalf of a Human Future*. New York: Teachers College Press.

Borer, K. T., Edington, D. W., & White, T. P. (Eds.). (1983). *Frontiers of Exercise Biology*. Champaign, IL: Human Kinetics.

Brock, D. H. (Ed.). (1984). *The Culture of Biomedicine: Studies in Science and Culture* (Vol. 1). Newark, DE: University of Delaware Press.

Bursch, R. (Ed.) (1990). *For Fun and Profit*. Philadelphia, PA: Temple University Press.

Butts, N. K., Gushiken, T. T., & Zarins, Bertram (Eds.). (1985). *The Elite Athlete*. Champaign, IL: Human Kinetics.

Chernin, K. (1985). *The Hungry Self: Women Eating and Identity*. New York: Times Books.

Clarke, D. H., & Eckert, H. M. (Eds.). (1985). *Limits of Human Performance*. Champaign, IL: Human Kinetics.

Dohesty, W. J., & Campbell, T. L. (1988). *Families and Health*. Beverly Hills, CA: Sage.

Drowatsky, J. N., & Armstrong, C. W. (1984). *Career Perspectives and Professional Foundations*. Englewood Cliffs, NJ: Prentice-Hall.

Eagleton, T. (1991). *Ideology: An Introduction*. New York: Vess.

Eichstaedt, C. B., & Lavay, B. W. (1992). *Physical Activity for Individuals With Mental Retardation*. Champaign, IL: Human Kinetics.

Ellis, M. J. (1988). *The Business of Physical Education*. Champaign, IL: Human Kinetics.

Freire, P. (1985). *The Politics of Education: Culture, Power, and Liberation*. Westport, CT: Bergin and Garvey.

Gerson, R. F. (1989). *Marketing Health/Fitness Services*. Champaign, IL: Human Kinetics.

Giroux, H. A. (1981). *Ideology, Culture, and the Process of Schooling*. London: Falmer Press.

Goodlad, J. L. (1984). *A Place Called School: Prospects for the Future*. New York: McGraw-Hill.

Graham, G., & Peron, M. (Eds.) (1985). *Sport Pedagogy*. Champaign, IL: Human Kinetics.

Hall, L. K. (Ed.). (1993). *Developing and Managing Cardiac Rehabilitation Programs*. Champaign, IL: Human Kinetics.

Hamill, J. (Ed.). (1992). *The Physically Challenged Child*. Champaign, IL: Human Kinetics.

Harrington, A. (1987). *Medicine, Mind, and the Double Brain*. Princeton, NJ: Princeton University Press.

Haynes, E. M., & Wells, C. L. (1986). *Environment and Human Performance*. Champaign, IL: Human Kinetics.

Hellison, D. R., & Templin, T. J. (1991). *A Reflective Approach to Teaching Physical Education*. Champaign, IL: Human Kinetics.

Hiatt, H. H. (1987). *America's Health in the Balance: Choice or Change*. New York: Harper and Row.

Hoberman, J. M. (1992). *Mortal Engines: The Science of Performance and the Dehumanization of Sport*. New York: Free Press.

Horn, T. S. (Ed.). (1992). *Advances in Sport Psychology*. Champaign, IL: Human Kinetics.

Illich, I. (1976). *Medical Nemesis: The Expropriation of Health*. New York: Pantheon.

Janeway, E. (1980). *Powers of the weak*. New York: A. A. Knopf.

Kaneke, M. (Ed.). (1990). *Fitness for the Aged, Disabled, and Industrial Worker*. Champaign, IL: Human Kinetics.

Kantes, R. M., (1983). *The Change Masters*. New York: Simon and Schuster.

Kirk, D., & Tinning, R. (Eds.) (1990). *Physical Education, Curriculum, and Culture: Critical Issues in the Contemporary Crisis*. London: Falmer.

Kohn, A. (1986). *No Contest: The Case Against Competition*. Boston: Houghton Mifflin.

Landers, D. M. (Ed.). (1986). *Sport and Elite Performers*. Champaign, IL: Human Kinetics.

Ludmerer, K. M. (1985). *Learning to Heal: The Development of American Medical Education*. New York: Basic Books.

Marshall, J. (1984). *Women Managers: Travelers in a Male World*. Chichester, England: John Wiley and Sons.

Morrison, M., White, R. P., & Van Velsor, E. (1987). *Breaking the Glass Ceiling*. Don Mills, Ontario: Addison-Wesley.

Mullin, B. J., Hardy, S., & Sutton, W. A. (1993). *Sport Marketing*. Champaign, IL: Human Kinetics.

Naisbitt, J., & Aburdene, P. (1985). *Reinventing the Corporation: Transforming Your Job and Your Company for the New Information Society*. New York: Warner Books.

Navarro, V. (1986). *Crisis, Health and Medicine: A Social Critique*. New York: Tavistock.

Numbers, R. L. (Ed.). (1980). *The Education of American Physicians*. Berkeley, CA: University of California Press.

O'Donnel, M. P., & Ainsworth, T. H. (1984). *Health Promotion in the Workplace*. New York: John Wiley.

Parks, J. B., & Zanger, B. R. K. (Eds.). (1990). *Sport and Fitness Management*. Champaign, IL: Human Kinetics.

Patton, R. W., Corry, J. M., Gettman, L. R., & Graf, J. S. (1986). *Implementing Health/Fitness Programs*. Champaign, IL: Human Kinetics.

Patton, R. W., Grantham, W. C., Gerson, R. F., & Gettman, L. R. (Eds.). (1989). *Developing and Managing Health/Fitness Facilities*. Champaign, IL: Human Kinetics.

Pearl, A. J. (Ed.). (1993). *The Athletic Female*. Champaign, IL: Human Kinetics.

Rink, J. E. (1985). *Teaching Physical Education for Learning*. St. Louis: Times Mirror/Mosby.

Sanders, S. W. (1992). *Designing Preschool Movement Programs*. Champaign, IL: Human Kinetics.

Schoeder, S. (Ed.). *Ecobehavioral Analysis and Developmental Disabilities*. New York: Springer-Verlag.

Shephard, R. J. (1990). *Fitness in Special Populations*. Champaign, IL: Human Kinetics.

Spirduso, W. W., & Eckert, H. M. (Eds.). (1989). *Physical Activity and Aging*. Champaign, IL: Human Kinetics.

Starr, P. (1982). *The social Transformation of American Medicine: The Rise of a Sovereign Profession and the Making of a Vast Industry*. New York: Basic Books.

Staudohar, P. (1986). *The Sports Industry and Collective Bargaining*. Ithaca, NY: Cornell University Press.

Suzuki, D. (1989). *Inventing the Future: Reflections on Science Technology and Nature*. Toronto, Ontario, Canada; Stoddart Publishing Co.

Templin, T. J., & Schempp, P. G. (Eds.). (1989). *Learning to Teach*. Indianapolis: Benchmark Press.

Wells, C. L. (1991). *Women, Sport, and Performance*. Champaign, IL: Human Kinetics.

William, M. H. (1989). *Beyond Training*. Champaign, IL: Human Kinetics.

Winnick, J. P. (Ed.) (1990). *Adapted Physical Education and Sport*. Champaign, IL: Human Kinetics.

Wright, W. (1982). *The Social logic of Health*. New Brunswick, NJ: Rutgers University Press.

# INDEX